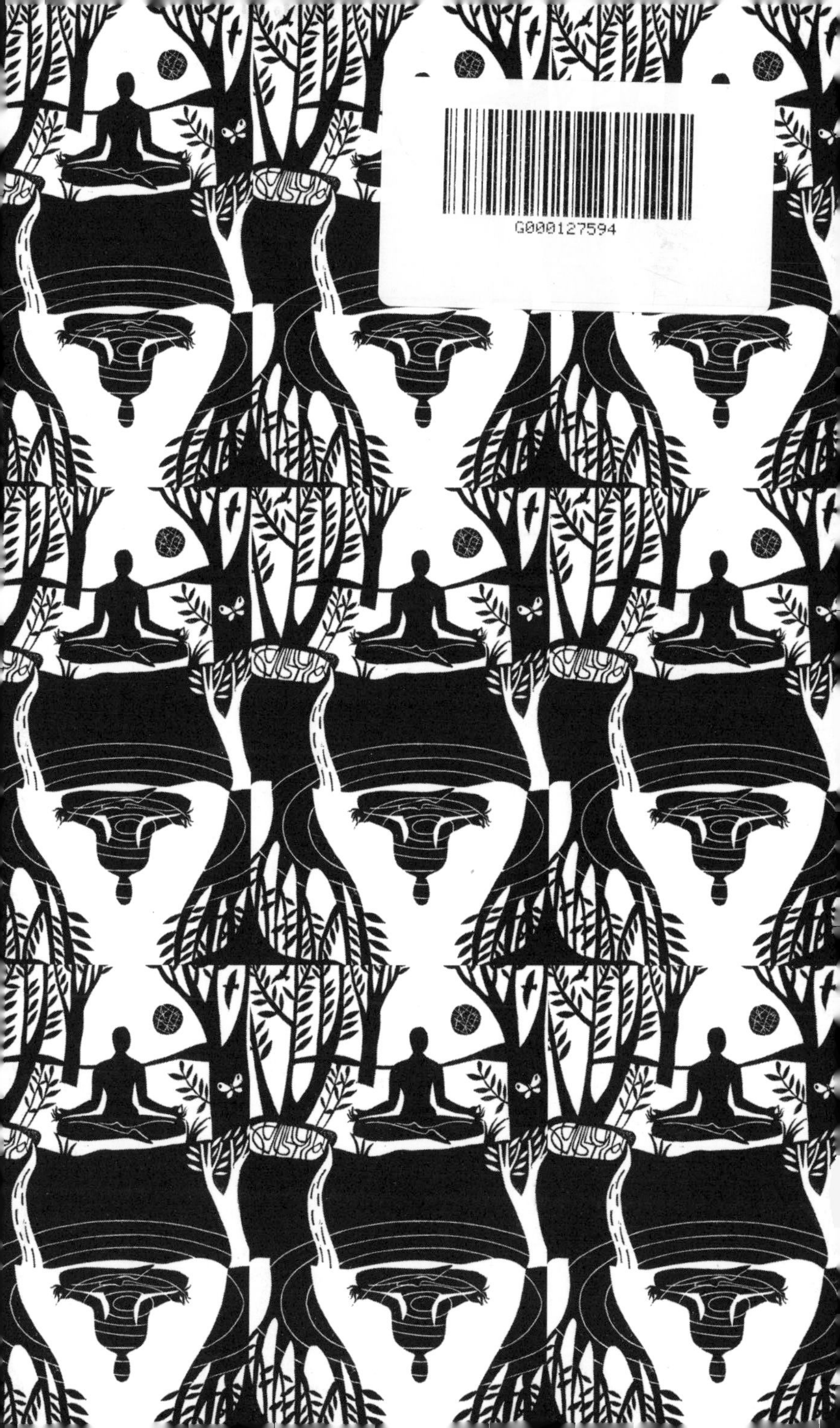

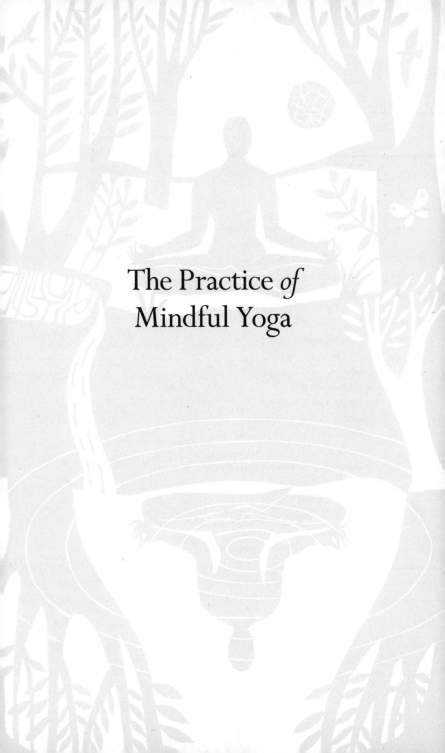

The Practice *of* Mindful Yoga

OTHER TITLES IN THIS SERIES:-

The Art of Mindful Baking

The Art of Mindful Birdwatching

The Art of Mindful Gardening

The Art of Mindful Silence

The Art of Mindful Singing

The Art of Mindful Walking

Einstein and the Art of Mindful Cycling

Galileo and the Art of Ageing Mindfully

Happiness and How it Happens

The Heart of Mindful Relationships

The Joy of Mindful Writing

The Mindful Art of Wild Swimming

Mindful Crafting

The Mindful Man

Mindful Pregnancy and Birth

Mindfulness and Compassion

Mindfulness and Music

Mindfulness and Surfing

Mindfulness and the Art of Drawing

Mindfulness and the Art of Managing Anger

Mindfulness and the Art of Urban Living

Mindfulness and the Journey of Bereavement

Mindfulness and the Natural World

Mindfulness at Work

Mindfulness for Black Dogs and Blue Days

The Mindfulness in Knitting

Zen and the Path of Mindful Parenting

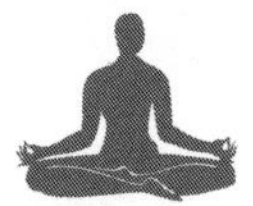

The Practice *of* Mindful Yoga

A Connected Path to Awareness

Hannah Moss

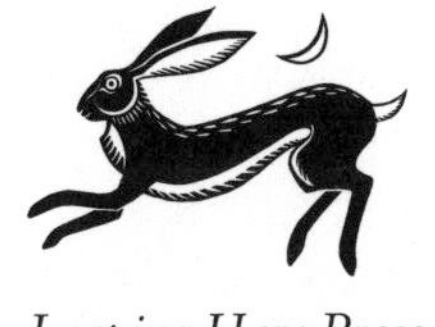

Leaping Hare Press

First published in the UK and North America in 2018 by

Leaping Hare Press

An imprint of The Quarto Group
The Old Brewery, 6 Blundell Street
London N7 9BH, United Kingdom
T (0)20 7700 6700 **F** (0)20 7700 8066
www.QuartoKnows.com

British Library Cataloguing-in-Publication Data
A catalogue record for this book is available from the British Library

ISBN: 978-1-78240-569-6

This book was conceived, designed and produced by

Leaping Hare Press

58 West Street, Brighton BN1 2RA, United Kingdom

Publisher Susan Kelly
Creative Director Michael Whitehead
Art Director James Lawrence
Editorial Director Tom Kitch
Commissioning Editor Monica Perdoni
Project Editor Elizabeth Clinton
Design Manager Anna Stevens
Designer Ginny Zeal
Illustrator Melvyn Evans

Printed in Slovenia by GPS Group

1 3 5 7 9 10 8 6 4 2

Contents

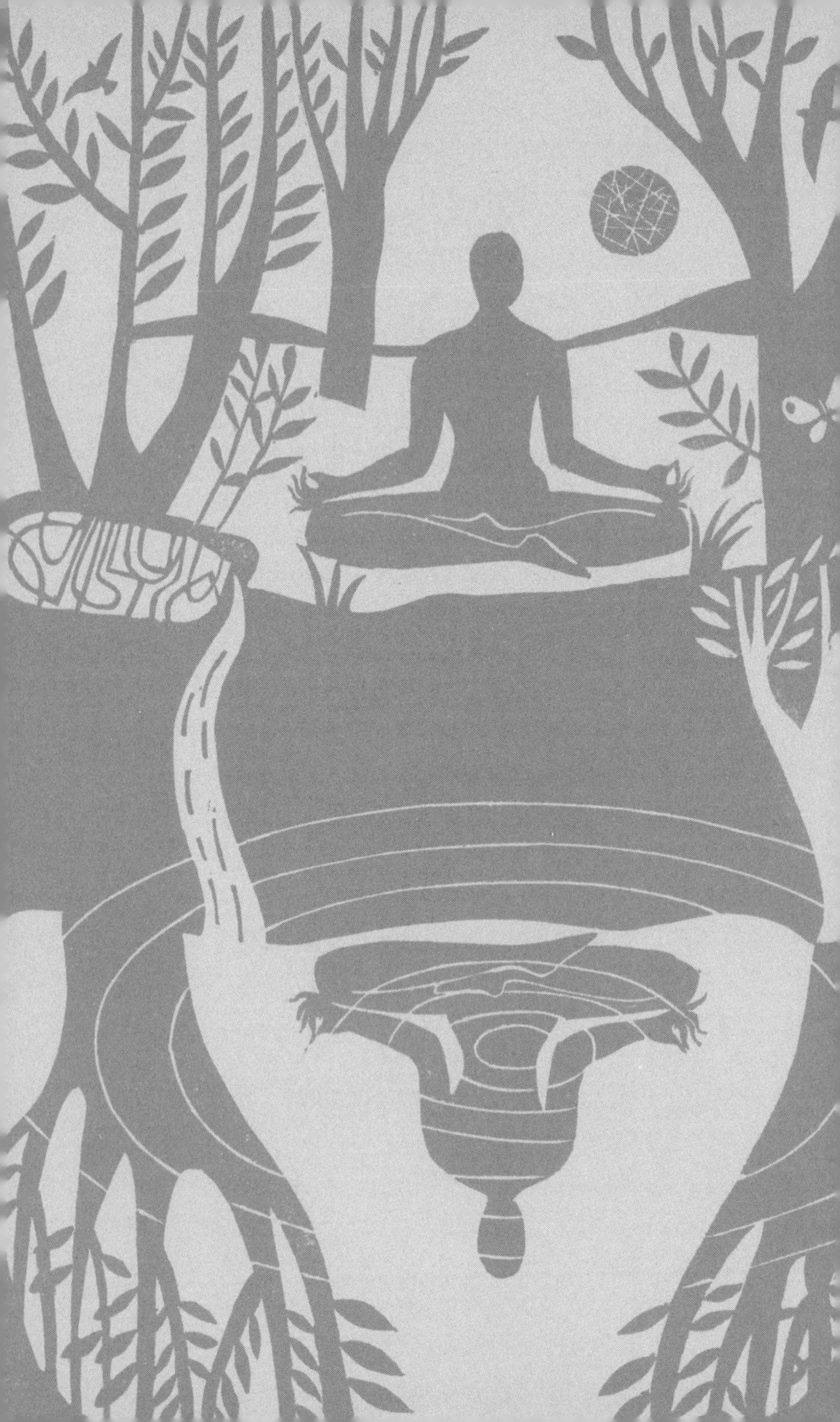

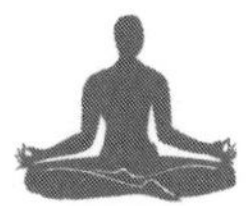

INTRODUCTION

Like most people, you have probably heard of yoga, even if you have never stepped onto a yoga mat. But have you ever considered the concept of mindful yoga and the many ways it could support the challenges faced in your life? My own yoga journey has so far spanned twenty years, and has transformed my mind and body in more ways than even I probably realize. However, it has only been comparatively recently that I have discovered the true meaning of mindful yoga, and how mindfulness can bring an even deeper level of awareness to your yoga practice.

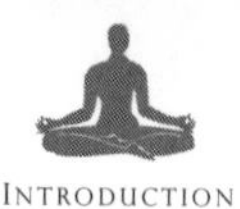

MY OWN YOGA JOURNEY

I remember the peace and tranquility I felt in my first few yoga classes, and how much I enjoyed moving my body. I had a sense of being given permission to go quietly within and not have to interact with anyone else. I was intrigued by the inner calm I felt, despite not really knowing, at the age of nineteen, what inner calm was.

I HAVE PRACTISED LOTS OF HATHA and Iyengar yoga over the years but for six years I had a daily 'Mysore-style' Ashtanga yoga practice. Essentially, this consisted of getting up at five a.m., heading to my local *shala* (traditional yoga studio) and sweating out a dynamic, two-hour practice before dashing off to work – six days a week, every week, for six years. It was intense and life-changing. But after so many years of committed daily practice, something eventually changed.

Losing the Connection

The best word I can find to describe how my practice had come to feel is 'mechanical'. I was still rolling out my mat each morning and completing my practice, but I was simply going through the motions. I had lost touch with the essence of yoga and why I had started practising in the first place. It had become a rigid part of my life, and an unnecessary pressure – something I 'should' do each morning, as it was part of who I was, it defined me. I was trying to fit the rest of my life around my yoga practice, rather than letting my yoga practice support the rest of my life.

What I realized most of all was that my mind was no longer present. Rather than bringing focused awareness onto my mat, I was actually practising 'mindless yoga'. I was not listening to my body. I had lost the union between mind, body and soul that is the very essence of yoga.

So I stopped. After six years of dedicating my life to this practice, I simply stopped. I found myself gravitating towards gentler, less dynamic yoga classes and tried many different styles and teachers, searching for something that felt right.

Discovering Mindful Yoga

And then I found it. I attended a new class taught by an experienced, local teacher and was blown away. There was no set sequence to follow, no 'full posture' to achieve, or correct count to master. There was simply the teacher's voice encouraging us to listen within and to pay attention to how our bodies felt.

At first, I did not understand the instructions. Where should my foot be? How should I move this arm? What shape should I be making? Then I realized it did not matter. This teacher was offering me a new way to see my practice. I was being given permission to move how I wanted to, how my body needed to. It was no longer about how the yoga looked from the outside; it was about how it felt from the inside.

And I discovered the very thing that had been missing in my yoga practice: mindfulness.

Why I Have Written This Book

Many would say that yoga today is a far cry from its Indian origins, as it gains more and more exposure around the world. We want to stretch our bodies to counteract our increasingly sedentary lifestyles. We want to switch off from all the screens and technology. We want to go within to escape the noise of our busy, modern lives – temporarily, at least.

Yoga is only safe and effective when it has mindfulness at its heart

There are so many styles of yoga, taught by thousands of individuals with vastly differing teaching styles. Yoga is becoming big business, with a myriad of classes, workshops, holidays, retreats, training events and online courses to choose from, not to mention the vast array of yoga clothes, books, mats, props, equipment and accessories on offer.

But I believe underlying all of this, regardless of which style you practise, where you practise or who you practise with, there is only one thing that really matters when it comes to yoga, and that is mindfulness.

I believe that yoga should always be practised mindfully. Yoga is only safe and effective when it has mindfulness at its heart. Mindless yoga is simply a form of exercise, whereas mindful yoga embodies the essence of yoga itself: union.

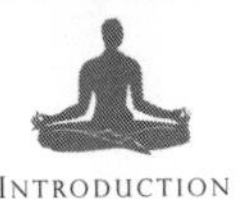

It is about uniting yoga and mindfulness into one seamless, conscious practice.

Is This Book for You?

My intention is that beginners and experienced practitioners alike will be able to benefit from the ideas shared in this book. If you are already familiar with yoga, perhaps you will be able to invite a more mindful presence into your existing practice. If you are new to yoga, I encourage you to appreciate the importance of bringing mindfulness into your practice right from the start.

The mindful practices outlined in this book are intended to form part of a yogic lifestyle that can be extended into everyday existence. I hope that this will encourage you to start allowing more awareness, more patience and more compassion into every area of your life – your relationships, work, social life, leisure activities, and of course, your yoga practice.

I do not claim to be an 'expert' in either yoga or mindfulness – indeed, by their very nature, these are not arts to be mastered, but lifelong practices to maintain. I hope, though, that by sharing what I have learned over the years and inviting you on this journey of self-discovery, you might feel inspired to find your own path.

The practice of mindful yoga has the power to lead us all on a conscious path to joyful, compassionate awareness. Are you ready to get connected?

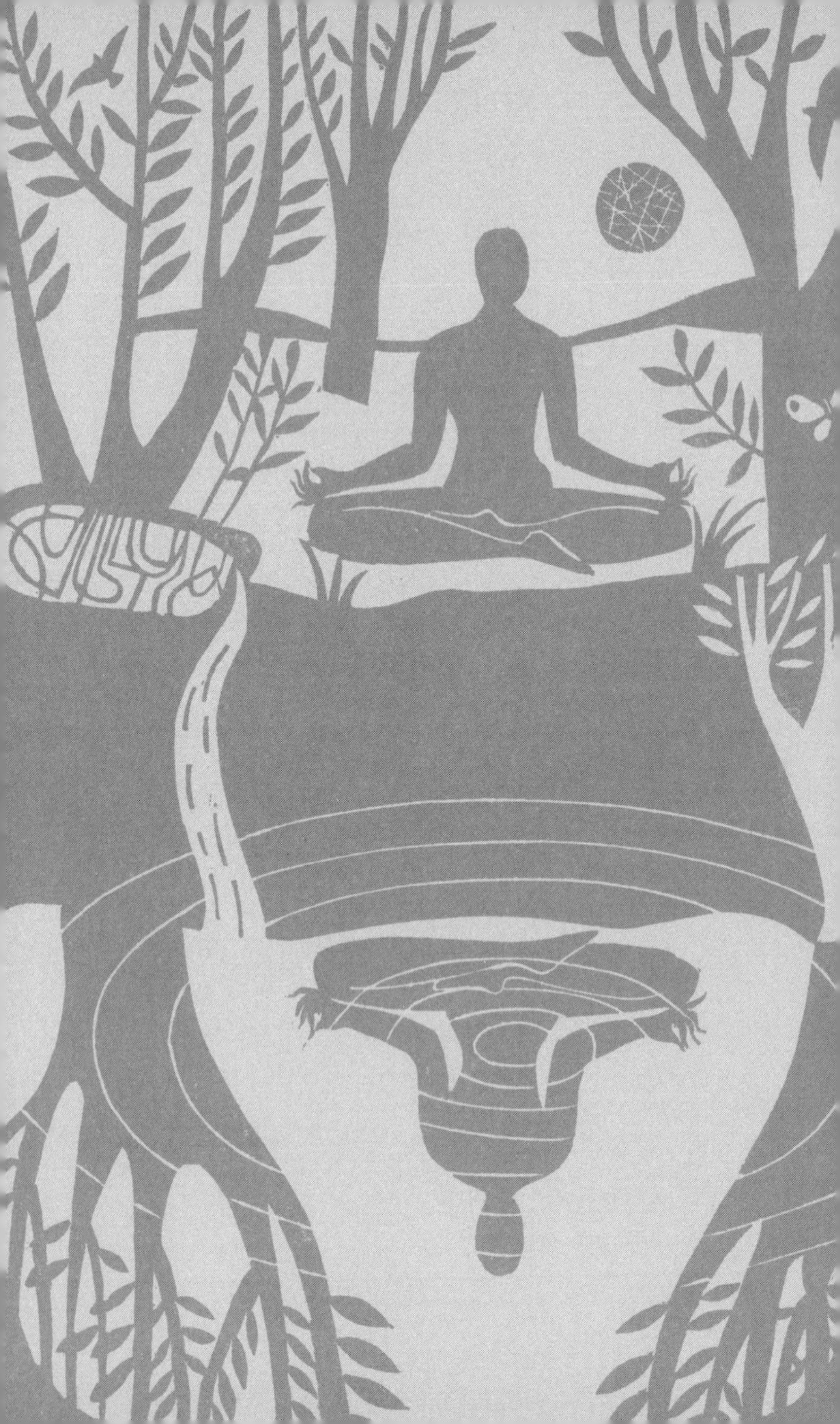

CHAPTER ONE

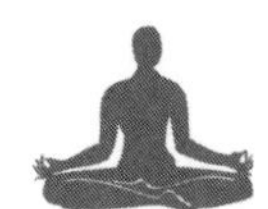

WHAT IS MINDFUL YOGA?

Yoga and mindfulness are both complex and subtle subjects. To help gain a clearer perspective, we will explore different interpretations and philosophies within the traditions of yoga, and from there, introduce mindfulness, considering what it means, whether you are a beginner or an advanced practitioner. With this understanding, mindfulness can be a tool for transformation, bringing lasting positive change into your life.

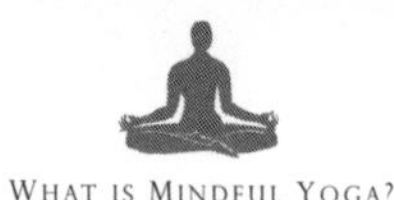

The Meaning of Yoga

Different cultures across the world offer a vast array of interpretations when it comes to the question, 'What is yoga?' Even if you asked two people from the same school or tradition, you would likely receive two very different answers. But there do seem to be some common uniting threads running through most of these interpretations as to what lies at the heart of yoga.

It is generally accepted that yoga is a combination of physical, mental and spiritual practices, which focus on strength, flexibility and breath control to improve overall wellbeing. The bodily postures, breathing techniques and simple meditation are commonly used for health and relaxation purposes.

While yoga is such an ancient art that its precise origins are not known, the best evidence we have suggests that it started out in ancient India around two to five thousand years ago.

Etymology

In Sanskrit the word yoga comes from the root *yuj*, which means 'to yoke' or 'to attach'. Therefore, the most common definition of yoga is 'union'. This has been interpreted as the union between the ego-self and the divine self; union with God; union of mind, body and soul; and union of the individual consciousness with the universal consciousness.

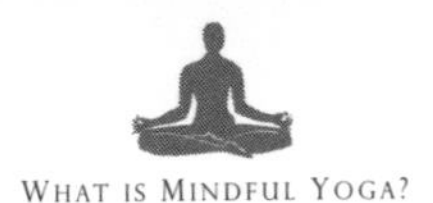

Another, similar, interpretation of yoga is integration – between mind and body, and between our outer and inner worlds. Many would say that the real purpose of yoga – instead of focusing purely on the form – is to embody this principle of integration in your practice.

Yoga as a Spiritual Practice

Yoga is commonly thought of as a physical practice: many view it as a way of bending and stretching the body and nothing more. However, the physical postures are only one aspect of yoga, known as *asana*. And as R. Sharath Jois said in a conference I attended in Mysore, India, in March 2014, 'Knowing only asana is like having a vehicle but not knowing how to drive it.'

One of the key elements of any yoga practice is the breath – indeed, the union of yoga also applies to the union of breath and movement. Unless you are practising a specific type of *pranayama,* or breath control exercise, it is important never to hold your breath during yoga but to inhale and exhale in harmony with your body's movements. Keeping this connection going is what sets yoga apart: if you are not linking breath with movement then it is not yoga, it is merely physical exercise.

If you are not linking breath with movement then it is not yoga, it is merely physical exercise

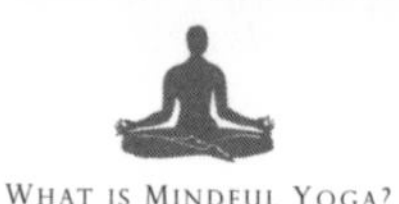

Mindful yoga is not about bending your body into a pretzel. In fact, it really does not matter what you do on your mat, as long as you are getting on it in the first place. There are no goals in yoga; there is nowhere to progress; there is nothing to be achieved. It is about the journey, not the destination. You could practise advanced postures every day for the rest of your life, but if you never meet your true self, never find peace within and are not able to live a happier, more aware existence, then what is the point?

If you can let go of the grasping and the attachment to goals, this is when real transformation can happen. It is about turning up, going through the process, facing yourself and dealing with your own personal challenges.

Mindful yoga is primarily a spiritual discipline, connecting our body, our breath and our mind so that we can turn our attention inwards and start getting to know ourselves a little better. We can learn to identify our habitual patterns and negative thought processes, making ourselves more aware of our experiences in the present moment.

Although yoga is a spiritual practice, you do not need to be religious in order to practise it. I think in the West the term 'spiritual' has become synonymous with 'other-worldly', belonging to another dimension. To my mind, spirituality simply means 'of spirit'. As human beings we are all made of, or have, spirit within us. Therefore, a spiritual practice is actually a *human* practice. It is anything you choose it to be – reading, writing, gardening, knitting, cycling, swimming, drawing, painting or yoga, for example. What makes it a spiritual practice rather than simply an activity, is bringing awareness to it. If it is something you do regularly, with intention, and with mindfulness, then I would argue that it is a spiritual practice.

What is Mindfulness?

In order to understand how to practise yoga more mindfully, it is important to first understand what mindfulness actually is. A brief introduction is included here, and in chapter three you will find a detailed explanation of some common mindful practices.

Mindfulness is a way of training yourself to focus on whatever is happening in the present moment. It can be thought of as paying attention, on purpose, in the present moment, without judgement.

As the pressures of modern life in our digital age increase, mindfulness is rapidly emerging as one of our most useful resources. The ability to bring more awareness into our lives and to ground ourselves in the present moment helps us to avoid being sucked back into the past or catapulted into the future. Even schools, prisons and government institutions in many countries are recognizing what an invaluable tool mindfulness can be.

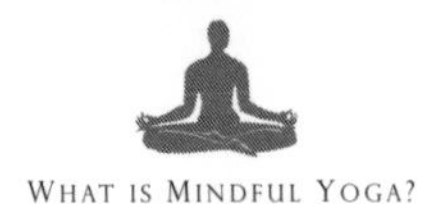

Blending East & West

Mindfulness has its roots in Buddhism. The *Satipatthana Sutta* – the *Discourse on the Foundations of Mindfulness* – is considered one of the most important texts of the ancient Theravadan tradition. In the East, mindfulness and meditation have existed as Buddhist practices for nearly three thousand years, and during the last two centuries these ideas have also spread to the West.

One of the key figures responsible for increasing the popularity of mindfulness in the West in recent years is Jon Kabat-Zinn. Originally a molecular biologist, he gave up his scientific career when he discovered Zen meditation and yoga, as he wanted to see if he could use these practices to treat sick patients. He founded a program called Mindfulness-Based Stress Reduction (MBSR) and has achieved remarkable results from teaching mindfulness meditation to people suffering with stress, chronic illness and pain.

Benefits of Mindfulness

It is generally thought that mindfulness can lead to a longer and healthier life. There is a growing body of scientific evidence that shows that regular mindfulness meditation offers many benefits, including:

- Increased concentration, memory and physical stamina
- Relief from anxiety and depression
- Reduced chronic pain, even from cancer

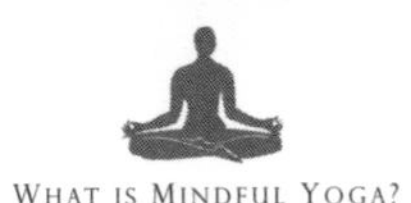

- Increased immunity to colds, flu and other diseases
- Relief from stressors leading to high blood pressure and heart disease
- Increased feelings of happiness, positivity and contentment

Consider how much suffering and conflict in the world is caused by people's reactions to their emotions: hurt, anger, frustration, pessimism, anxiety, depression, loneliness. If everyone could learn to use mindfulness to deal with their reactions to these emotions in a better way, I truly believe the world would be a more harmonious place.

Practising Mindfulness

Two of the key elements of mindfulness are awareness and compassion. Awareness simply means becoming aware – not only of the present moment, but also of our own thought processes, behaviours and reactions. Rather than trying to change external circumstances that are out of our control, we simply try to become aware of our response to them. As humans, we all experience suffering; it is inevitable. With mindfulness we are not trying to escape from suffering, but improve our relationship to it.

For example, you might be walking down the street and someone pushes past and knocks into you. It is very likely that your initial reaction is one of annoyance, frustration or even rage. How dare they knock into you? Why didn't they look where they were going? They should have been more careful.

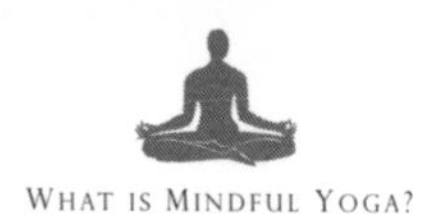

Perhaps you often react like this and find yourself feeling angry with other people.

If you are able to practise mindfulness in these moments, you might find that you start to see things differently. You might wonder what was going on for the other person. Why were they in a hurry? Perhaps a loved one has been in an accident, or their partner is about to give birth. Maybe they are late for a job interview and feeling very stressed. Probably they did not mean to knock into you and felt bad for doing so, but did not have time to stop and apologize. Perhaps you would do the same if you were in their shoes.

With mindfulness we are not trying to escape from suffering, but improve our relationship to it

So, this is also where compassion comes in: stopping to think about what is going on for the other person in the situation. Can you stop and breathe for a moment, become aware of how you are feeling, and think kindly of the other person? You might realize that getting worked up is actually counter-productive, and the only person it will ultimately affect is you!

One of the key aspects of mindfulness is being able to bring your attention to the present moment. If we are fully present in this moment, then we cannot be worrying about the past or fearing the future. We are only engaged with what is happening right now: what we can see, hear, taste, smell and feel.

MINDFUL EXERCISE

AWAKENING THE SENSES

This exercise can be practised at any time of day, no matter where you are or what you are doing. It is the perfect tool for when you feel stressed, overwhelmed or agitated, as it will bring your mind away from your negative thoughts and into the present moment.

1. As soon as you realize you are lost in your thoughts or feeling stressed, simply stop what you are doing and bring yourself into the present moment. Close your eyes and take a deep breath.

2. Now, open your eyes and look around you. Notice five things you can see.

3. Really look at each object, and try to note some of the details, for example, 'I can see a roof with red tiles' or 'I can see that elderly woman with a walking stick heading towards me.'

4. Now, open your ears and notice five things you can hear. Again, include some details, for example,'I can hear a siren wailing in the distance' or 'I can hear the floorboards creaking in the next room.' Take time to fully listen and observe the quality of these different sounds.

5. Finally, notice five things you can feel. These could be inside or outside of your body, for example, 'I can feel my breath as I exhale through my nose' or 'I can feel the fabric of my socks against my feet.' Again, pay attention to how these things feel to you.

By focusing your attention on what you can see, hear and feel in the present moment, you are cultivating a crucial point of awareness. This is the very essence of mindfulness. You should find that your mind becomes a little clearer and you feel a little calmer.

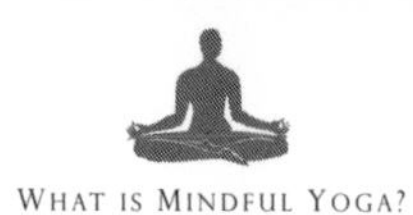

AN INTRODUCTION TO YOGA PHILOSOPHY

To give us a better insight into the history and development of yoga, it is useful to take a look at some of the philosophy behind it. This helps us to understand yoga as a spiritual practice, and see how we might use mindfulness to apply the yogic principles to our own lives for a more rewarding, enriching experience.

THERE ARE MANY HINDU SCRIPTURES and texts involved in yogic philosophy. These are composed primarily in the ancient Indian language Sanskrit and include the *Vedas*, the *Upanishads*, the *Puranas* and the *Bhagavad Gita*. However, there are two key texts that refer specifically to the practice of modern yoga. These are the *Hatha Yoga Pradipika* and the *Yoga Sutras of Patañjali*.

Hatha Yoga Pradipika

The *Hatha Yoga Pradipika* (meaning 'Light on Hatha Yoga') was written in Sanskrit by Swami Svatmarama in the fifteenth century. It is considered one of the most influential surviving manuals on Hatha yoga.

Hatha yoga was developed in India and consists of physical postures, or asana practice, as well as a focus on breathing, a good diet and exercises to purify the body and mind.

It is said that most forms of yoga were originally developed from Hatha yoga, which was revived by yoga teacher Tirumalai

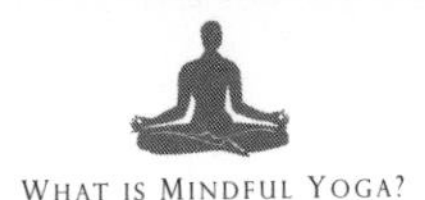

Krishnamacharya (1888–1989) in the 1920s. He inspired many of his students to develop different forms of yoga, all based on his method, and these students later went on to become renowned teachers. Among them were B.K.S. Iyengar, who developed Iyengar yoga, and K. Pattabhi Jois, who developed Ashtanga Vinyasa yoga. There are also many other styles of yoga that have developed from Hatha, including: Kundalini yoga, which involves the awakening of *kundalini* energy through the subtle body channels; Bikram yoga in which a set series of postures is practised in a heated room; and Kripalu yoga, which considers your body as the centre of your being, and therefore your best teacher.

The *Hatha Yoga Pradipika* includes information about the various types of bodily postures (asanas), breath control (pranayama), body locks (*bandhas*), symbolic gestures (*mudras*), energy centres (*chakras*) and meditation.

Patañjali's Yoga Sutras

The *Yoga Sutras of Patañjali* is an ancient text written in Sanskrit by Sage Patañjali some time around the fourth or fifth century. It consists of 196 *sutras* (aphorisms or statements) setting out the principles of yoga.

Scholars have always considered the *Yoga Sutras of Patañjali* to be one of the foundations of Hindu classical yoga philosophy. In the twentieth century it became more widely known among yoga practitioners in the West.

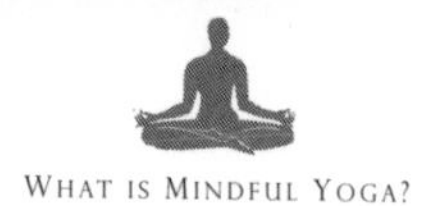

The Purpose of Yoga

In the second sutra of chapter one of Patañjali's *Yoga Sutras*, he defines the meaning of yoga as *yogas citta vritti nirodhah*. There are many interpretations of this sutra, but it is generally translated as, 'Yoga is the stilling of the modifications of the mind.' This term *citta vritti* is often referred to as 'mind chatter' or 'monkey mind'. Therefore, according to Patañjali, one of the goals of yoga is to control and calm this monkey mind, thereby reducing stress and increasing self-awareness. This is why it is often reported that the purpose of yoga is to prepare the body for meditation.

As R. Sharath Jois put it during the 2014 Mysore conference I mentioned earlier, 'Mind is like monkey, jumping here and there. How to still that mind is called yoga.'

The Eight Limbs

In chapter two, Patañjali divides the practice of yoga into eight aspects. These are the principles that form the basis of Hatha yoga and also give Ashtanga yoga its name (Ashtanga literally means 'eight-limbed'). These eight components, in order, are:

1. *Yama* – ethical observances or principles
2. *Niyama* – internal commitments or guidelines
3. *Asana* – physical postures
4. *Pranayama* – breath control
5. *Pratyahara* – turning the attention inwards

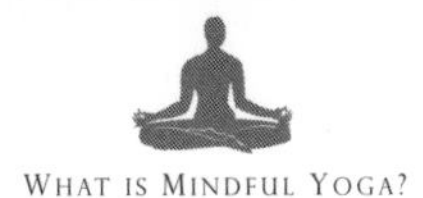

6. *Dharana* – concentration or focus
7. *Dhyana* – meditation or contemplation
8. *Samadhi* – union or oneness with the divine (often interpreted as enlightenment)

It is interesting to note the sequence in which Patañjali suggests approaching these limbs. The physical practice, asana, appears only third in the list, meaning there are other, more spiritual elements to be introduced into your life first in order to help with personal growth. Yama and niyama are the foundation of any mindful yoga practice, and without them there can be no success in meditation and no understanding of yoga in its wider sense.

THE FIVE YAMAS

There are five yamas listed in Patañjali's Yoga Sutras, which are a set of ethical observances or behaviours that govern how you relate to others. These should form the basis of how you live your life if you want to fully embrace all aspects of yoga and lead a more compassionate, fulfilling existence.

Ahimsa

The first yama says you should practice *ahimsa*, or non-violence. This means not causing harm to any living being, in any form, at any time, for any reason – in word, thought or deed. An example of ahimsa living can be seen in the vegetarianism followed by most dedicated yoga practitioners around the world. It also encompasses non-violence towards oneself, so practising self-kindness and self-compassion, which are also key elements of mindfulness. If you live your life in a non-violent way, then those around you will cease to be hostile.

Satya

Satya means truth, so this yama indicates that you should always tell the truth in thought, word and deed. However, this is not always as straightforward as it seems. If we consider this yama in conjunction with the first, it follows that the truth should be pleasant to others and not cause undue harm, so an unpleasant truth perhaps should not be told. It can also be applied to recognizing the truth within yourself. When you observe the chatterings, reactions and thought processes of your mind, you can learn to accept what you find and not lie to or deceive yourself.

Asteya

This yama refers to non-stealing, but does not only apply to theft; it also extends to not being envious of others, not manipulating others using false words, and not trying to achieve personal gain under the guise of truthfulness. If you are able to practise non-attachment (a lifelong practice indeed!), this is one of the best ways to counteract the desire to steal, compete or show off.

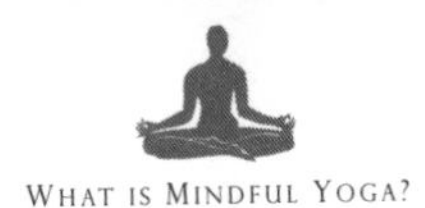

Brahmacharya

Brahmacharya has been interpreted as chastity, marital fidelity or sexual restraint. It is to do with moderation and abstinence; traditionally, sexual abstinence includes abstaining from masturbation, sexual thoughts and fantasies. In a simpler form, it could be interpreted as being loyal and faithful to a committed partner. It is also about preserving vital energy and using that energy in the right way. In the context of mindful yoga, perhaps this could be interpreted as being committed to your practice and leading a well-balanced life, refraining from misconduct, and taking everything in moderation.

Aparigraha

The final yama focuses on non-possessiveness or non-attachment. It says you should only take what you need, not be greedy, and not desire that which is superfluous to the physical body. When practising mindful yoga, it is wise to loosen your attachment to progression in your yoga practice and, rather than trying to 'get better at it', allow it to just be. In the same vein, don't try to change yourself or become someone different, but just accept yourself for who you are, in this moment, right now. This is a lot harder than it sounds but continued practice is the key.

Accept yourself for who you are, in this moment, right now

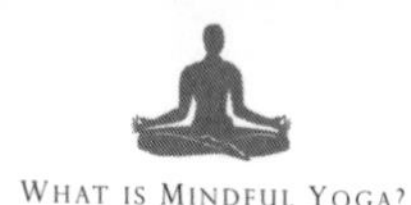

The Five Niyamas

The five niyamas outlined in Patañjali's Yoga Sutras are a set of commitments to yourself in order to enhance your personal growth and allow you to lead a more spiritual, or awakened, existence.

Sauca

Sauca means purity or clarity, and refers to speech, mind and body. In terms of speech, this can mean not using foul or offensive language. Healthy, positive thoughts will keep your mind pure, as will keeping a clear mind during your mindful yoga practice.

Keeping your body pure could mean eating only natural, healthy foods and using only natural, organic toiletries and cosmetics. Like many yogis around the world, I believe in the saying 'Your body is a temple'. The skin is the largest organ of the human body, and absorbs most substances into the bloodstream; therefore if you would not put something *in* your body, then why put it *on* your body?

Santosha

This niyama relates to contentment, and includes acceptance of others, acceptance of one's own circumstances and optimism. It also relates to finding happiness from within, which can be a lasting joy, rather than happiness from material things, which can only ever be temporary.

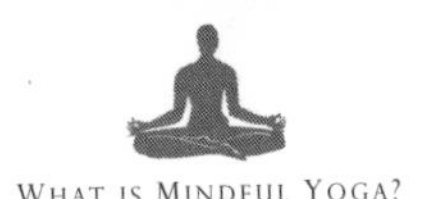

Acceptance is such an important theme in mindful yoga, because if you cannot accept where you are right now – both in your yoga practice and in your life – then you are probably grasping for something outside yourself. You may be wishing you were somewhere else, or that you would be happier if only you could touch your toes in that particular yoga posture. If you can find your way to completely accepting yourself for who you are, including whatever stage your yoga practice is at, the chances are you will start to see yourself and your circumstances more positively. A great way to do this is to start a gratitude practice (page 86).

Tapas

Tapas means persistence, perseverance or austerity. It relates to observing self-discipline and leading a life of principle. This includes following a disciplined diet, avoiding negative influences and keeping a steady spiritual practice. The line between dedication and obsession can be thin when it comes to yoga: you need a certain amount of discipline to keep getting on to your mat, but you do not want this to become a chore, a habit or an addiction. Ideally, you step onto your mat because you want to, because you know how good it makes you feel, not because you think you ought to or because you are on autopilot. If, like me, you are an expert at putting pressure on yourself to do the 'right' thing or to do what is expected of you, you need to be careful with this one!

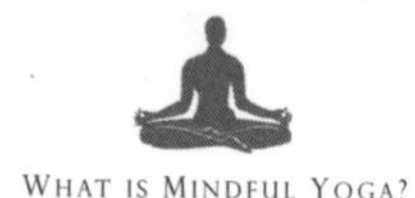

Swadhyaya

This niyama relates to self-study, and has been interpreted as gaining a deeper understanding of yoga, by studying yogic philosophy and the lessons we have absorbed from our teachers. It can also be thought of more generally as self-reflection and consideration of one's thoughts, speech and actions. *Swadhyaya* can be interpreted as thinking before you speak or act, asking yourself, 'Do I need to speak these words? Are they kind? Will my words or actions cause offence or harm to others? Does this thought need to be acted on, or is it best kept to myself?'

During your practice, or indeed during any moment of your day, you can also ask yourself, 'How am I feeling? What do my thoughts look like today? How are my moods? Does this posture feel different to the last time I practised it? What am I grateful for in this moment?' and so on. In so doing, you apply Swadhyaya to the continuous curiosity that is necessary in order to better understand yourself.

Ishvara Pranidhana

The final niyama refers to contemplation of Ishvara, meaning God or Supreme Being, in order to gain deeper spiritual knowledge. Even if you have no religious affiliations or beliefs, you could still apply this concept to anything that has significance for you, for example, the universe, love, life or even your true self.

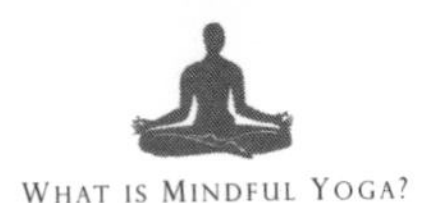

You might feel like dedicating your mindful yoga practice to a particular deity or symbolic being, such as Buddha, Ganesha (the Hindu elephant god), Jesus or your angels. You could also dedicate your practice to anyone important in your life, such as a partner, family member, close friend, beloved pet or even a community, association or charity that is dear to you. Making a dedication in this way is a wonderful way to start your practice and help you feel connected to others.

Elements of Yoga Practice

There are many elements of yoga referenced in the Hatha Yoga Pradipika and the Yoga Sutras of Patañjali. Ideally, your yoga practice would include all of these elements, but in reality they are unlikely to be incorporated into every yoga session or class. Nonetheless, it is useful to understand what these elements are and the importance of each.

Asana

Asana is the name for the physical poses or postures in yoga. When most people think of or refer to yoga it is actually the asana practice they mean, whereas the true meaning of yoga goes far beyond merely the physical practice.

In Sanskrit, *asana* means 'sitting down' or 'to sit down' and in his *Yoga Sutras*, Patañjali defines asana as, 'to be seated in a position that is firm, but relaxed.' Hence, traditionally, asana

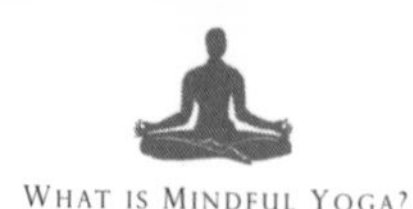

MINDFUL YOGA EXERCISE

YOGA ASANA: WARRIOR TWO (VIRABHADRASANA II)

Warrior Two is a strong standing posture that stretches and strengthens your legs, ankles, shoulders, chest and groin.

1. Stand at the front of your mat with your feet together. Inhale, then exhale and step out into a wide stance along your mat, with your arms out to the sides.

2. Turn your right foot out (so it is parallel with the long edge of your mat) and turn your left foot in slightly. The heel of your right foot should be in line with the arch of your left foot.

3. Bend your right knee so that it is aligned directly above your right ankle, sinking your hips towards the floor.

4. Try to feel whether your left arm is straight before looking to check. Then look towards your right hand.

5. Keep your tailbone tucked in, your feet grounded and your legs active – your thighs should be doing most of the work.

6. Take a few deep breaths, focusing your attention on the air as it travels in and out of your body.

7. Now take your attention to different areas. Are your shoulders relaxed and not scrunched up to your ears? How do your thighs feel? You might feel a strong, burning sensation in them. Can you take your breath there to help ease this?

8. Bring curiosity into your practice, but make sure any movements are made slowly and mindfully. You might feel like moving your arms, turning your neck or pulsing your hips up and down.

9. When you need to come out, push up strongly through your thighs on an inhalation and step to the front of your mat.

10. Repeat on the other side.

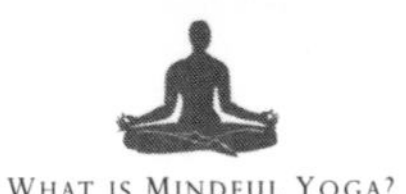

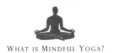

referred only to seated postures, but its usage has been extended to refer to all yoga poses.

Pranayama

Pranayama is a Sanskrit word meaning to control the *prana*, also known as the life force or breath. There are many different types of pranayama, or breathing exercises, involving the speed, quality and restriction of the breath.

Pranayama is the fourth limb of Patañjali's eight limbs of yoga (after asana) and many therefore believe it should not be introduced until a practitioner has established a solid asana practice, which could take several years. Traditionally speaking, you should only practise pranayama under the guidance of an experienced teacher. However, there are many simple breath exercises that can be incorporated into your mindful yoga practice from the beginning, and we shall explore these further in chapter two.

Bandha

The bandhas are thought of as body locks and are used to create energetic seals to keep prana contained. There are three main bandhas in the body:

- *Mula bandha* – contraction of the perineum, very similar to tightening the pelvic floor.
- *Uddiyana bandha* – contraction of the abdomen, similar to sucking in the belly.

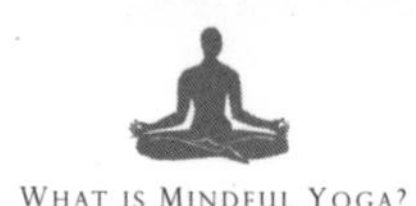

• *Jalandhara bandha* – contraction of the throat, made by tucking the chin into the chest.

The first two are the most common. If these are engaged during your yoga practice they can help to develop strong core muscles, which can aid with balancing and inverted postures and help to protect your lower back.

Drishti

Drishti means 'gazing point' in Sanskrit and is a way of developing concentrated intention in your mindful yoga practice.

In Ashtanga yoga, every asana has an associated drishti where you should focus your attention by holding your gaze on that body part, for example, the big toe, the tip of your nose or the tips of your fingers. This is to help keep your mind focused on the asana you are in, so you can concentrate on your breathing and avoid distractions.

Chakra

The chakras are energy centres in the body, which are referred to in many yogic texts and are often used in meditation, energy healing and martial arts.

There are seven chakras in the body located at the base of the spine, the sacrum, the navel, the heart, the throat, the third eye, and the crown. Each chakra has a specific colour and symbolism associated with it, and it is said that if one or more of your chakras becomes blocked, this can cause various

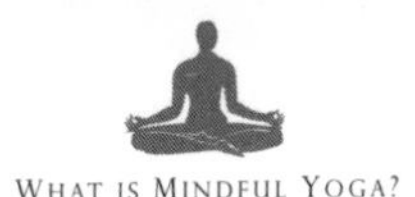

emotional, psychological and physical issues. Certain yoga postures can be used to cleanse, balance and open the chakras.

Mudra

A mudra is a symbolic gesture, most often made with the hands and fingers. In yoga, you usually use mudras while sitting in meditation or practising pranayama, to activate different parts of the body involved with breathing and to affect the flow of prana.

One of the simplest and most common mudras is the chin mudra. This is where you press the tips of your forefingers and thumbs together to form a circle, extend your remaining three fingers out straight, and place your hands palm up on your knees whilst sitting cross-legged or on a chair.

Mantra

A *mantra* is a chant or prayer that is repeated over and over for ritualistic or spiritual reasons. It is often said that the meaning of a mantra is less important than its resonance. The quality of the sound produced, and the feeling this evokes in the practitioner, is where the magic of a mantra lies. Mantras can be musically uplifting and spiritually meaningful and it has been argued that mantra meditation can help to induce an altered state of consciousness.

The simplest and most well known mantra is the word *Om* (or *Aum*). This has many different meanings for different traditions, but is generally translated as the sound of the soul, or the sound of the universe. It is the closest word in Sanskrit to 'yes' and is also interpreted as 'everything', so in a way we are saying yes to everything. It is often recited at the beginning and end of chapters in sacred Hindu and spiritual texts, before reciting prayers, at certain ceremonies and during meditation and yoga.

Chanting three Oms at the end of your mindful yoga sequence is a great way to close your practice. This is how many group yoga classes end, and we shall incorporate this into the end of our practice in the final chapter.

An Introduction to Mindful Yoga

Now that we have a better understanding of the benefits of yoga and mindfulness, we can consider how we might start to combine them into one seamless practice.

Mindful yoga is about bringing clarity and awareness into your yoga practice. It is about accepting where you are right now and listening to your body. Rather than copying what someone else is doing, or even strictly following a teacher's instructions, it is about practising in a way that is right for you.

Of course, I am not saying you should not follow a teacher; quite the contrary. I believe it is very important to find a

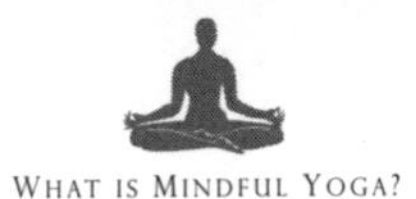

teacher that is right for you and to follow their guidance, particularly as a beginner. This will ensure you have a good foundation for your practice in terms of breathing, correct alignment and injury avoidance. But a good teacher will act only as a guide and will allow you to find your own way within your own practice. Once you become more familiar with the asanas and with different yoga styles, you can begin to modify and adapt them to suit your own mind and body. You can move into them in a way that is right for you; you can integrate different styles of yoga into your practice, and draw on your own experience and intuition.

There is a saying in yoga, 'Steady body, steady mind', but all too often the mind is not steady; it is too caught up in the ego, constantly comparing itself to others. You want to be a 'better' person, do 'better' postures, live a 'better' life. Mindfulness can be the antidote to the ego: grounding you in present moment experience, bringing you into the now, helping you to focus only on what you are feeling and experiencing right now, your bodily sensations, not getting caught up in the past or the future.

Over the next few chapters we will explore this practice more deeply. In the final chapter we will consolidate everything we have learned and discover how we can integrate these tools and techniques into one combined, invaluable practice for bringing real transformation into your life: the practice of mindful yoga.

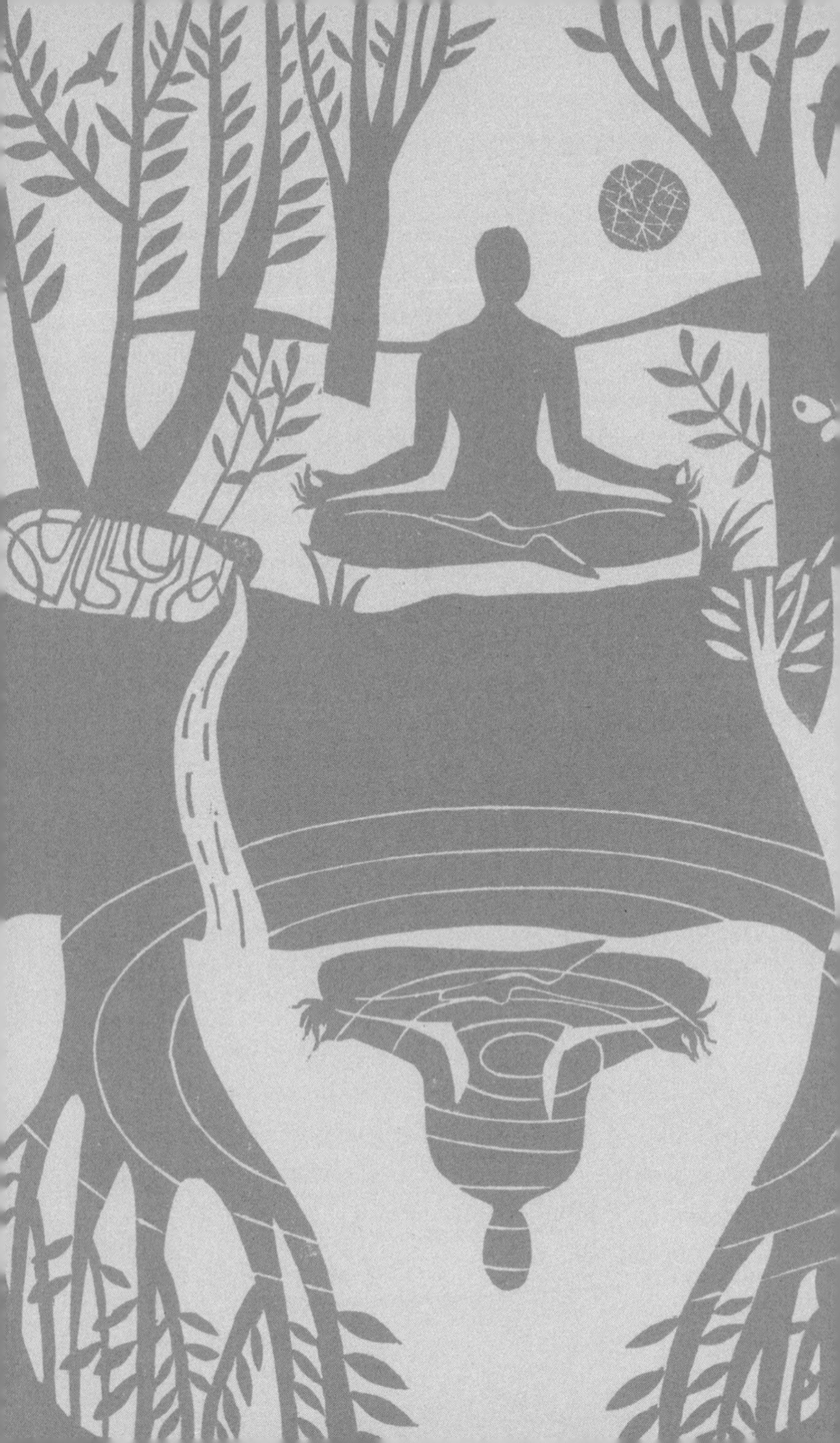

CHAPTER TWO

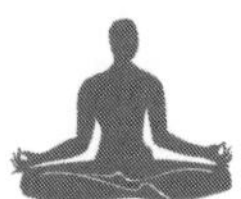

The Bridge Between Yoga & Mindfulness

Are mindfulness and yoga distinct practices? In my view, there is one tool that undeniably unites them, acting as a connecting bridge: the breath. Mindfulness meditation, just like yoga, is a practice of presence and awareness, using the breath to anchor the mind within the body.

INTRODUCTION TO THE BREATH

The breath is not something we usually pay much attention to. Inhaling and exhaling is part of being human, of being alive; it simply happens without us thinking about it. In fact, most of us probably take it for granted, even though we breathe around 20,000 times per day. But it is actually one of the most useful elements, if not the cornerstone, of any mindful yoga practice.

THE BREATH PLAYS A KEY ROLE in our moods and emotions. We can see this in expressions such as, 'Breathe a sigh of relief', 'Breathing down your neck', 'Takes your breath away', 'Breath of fresh air', and 'Take a few deep breaths'. When we are shocked, we may 'catch our breath' for a moment, and when we are relaxed, we breathe from our bellies. The rhythm of our breath also influences our perception: when it is fast and shallow, our vision narrows and we are less aware of our feelings; when it is calm and deep, there is more space to observe what is going on in the rest of our body, and we are more aware of our emotions and sensations.

But how often do we pause to notice what actually happens when we breathe – what happens physically, emotionally, mentally? Have you ever noticed, for instance, that when the air travels in through your nose or mouth, it is fairly cool, at room temperature, and when it leaves again it is warmer, at body temperature?

Observing the breath is a key aspect of both yoga and mindfulness because it grounds you in the here and now. The breath does not know past or future; it only exists in the present. Learning to harness and control the breath means we can use it to calm ourselves down, steady the body and still the mind.

If you walked into any Mysore-style Ashtanga yoga shala, the main sound you would hear would be the collective breath of the practitioners – all moving at different times, at their own pace, but all following the same sequence and all following the breath. This was one of the things that attracted me to the Ashtanga practice in the first place. Seeing a room full of people practising together, but following their own internal rhythm, and hearing only their breathing – it was truly mesmerizing.

The breath does not know past or future; it only exists in the present

The breath is the unifying tool between yoga and mindfulness. You cannot enter into either of these practices without at least being aware of the breath, if not fully integrating it into your practice. It is therefore essential to understand how to use the breath in mindful yoga, and we shall consider this more deeply in the succeeding sections. But first, let us take a closer look at mindfulness meditation, as this is an important partner to mindful yoga.

INTRODUCTION TO MINDFULNESS MEDITATION

Learning to meditate is intrinsically linked to learning the practice of mindful yoga. We cannot really understand one without first understanding the other. The most important things to remember when it comes to mindfulness meditation are: get comfortable; let go of pressure and pre-conceptions; keep it regular.

IT IS WIDELY BELIEVED THAT THE ORIGINAL PURPOSE of yoga was to prepare the body for meditation. I believe that yoga and meditation can work closely together and be mutually beneficial. By practising yoga regularly, we are able to bring more strength and flexibility into the body, which can help us to sit comfortably in meditation for longer periods. Similarly, a regular meditation practice can help to bring more clarity and compassion into all areas of our life, including yoga.

The more awareness we can bring to how our mind works, the more we can start to recognize our negative thought patterns and the points at which these are spiralling out of control, or taking us on an undesirable journey within our own minds.

What is Meditation?

In a nutshell, meditation is the primary, conscious path to achieving a state of mindfulness. It is a common misconception that meditation means emptying the mind. As any seasoned meditator will tell you, this is a near-impossible task! It is not possible to empty our mind, because our mind is full of thoughts. This is a simple neurological fact. However, what we can control is our reaction to those thoughts.

Very simply, meditation is a technique to calm and still the mind, but not necessarily empty it. It is about being rather than doing. The primary focus is to observe the thoughts that arise, but not engage with them, and instead to simply let them pass you by. Some people use visualization to help with this, for example, seeing your thoughts as clouds drifting by in the sky, as butterflies quietly fluttering past, or as balloons that you can gently pat away out of sight.

Meditation is the primary, conscious path to achieving a state of mindfulness

When we talk about meditation, we are usually referring to a formal practice. This generally involves sitting (or lying) quietly for a set amount of time, whilst focusing your attention on a single element of your consciousness, for example, the breath, your bodily sensations or the sounds around you.

Learning to Meditate

The great thing about meditation is that you need very few tools or pieces of equipment to get started. You can practise almost anywhere, whenever you have a few minutes to spare.

You could be at home, on the bus, or even waiting in a queue; no one needs to know that you are even doing it.

The best way to get started, though, is at home, where you can take time to make yourself comfortable and get 'in the zone'. In order to create optimal conditions for your practice, it is important to do a little preparation first:

- Find a quiet place where you will not be disturbed.
- Make sure you are free from distractions: close the door; turn off your phone; keep pets out of the room.
- Find a position you can comfortably stay in for the duration of your session. Contrary to popular belief, meditation is not meant to be torture. It does not need to be difficult or challenging, and feeling comfortable is actually a very important part of the practice. See 'Finding the Right Meditation Posture' for more detail on this.
- Make sure you will be warm enough for the duration of your practice. As you will be staying in one position for a while, your body temperature will drop, so you might want to put on warm clothes and wrap a blanket around yourself.
- Most people find closing their eyes during meditation helps them to stay more internally focused. However, if this does not feel right for you, or if you are feeling particularly drowsy, you can keep your eyelids half open and focus on a single point just in front of you.

Personally, I find it easiest to meditate early in the morning, before too many distractions of the day have kicked in. I turn

Finding the Right Meditation Posture

You can lie down to meditate, as long as there is no risk of you falling asleep. Make sure your back is fully supported and your head is not tipped back. You might want to keep your knees bent with your feet flat on the floor to release any tension in your lower back.

If you choose to sit, the most important thing to remember is to keep your back straight. If you are able to sit cross-legged, make sure you can stay upright without slouching. I would recommend sitting your buttocks on a cushion or yoga block. Make sure there is no strain on your knees and they are not lifting up off the floor. If they are, try raising your seat or placing a cushion underneath your knees to support them.

If you are unable to comfortably sit cross-legged, you might prefer to kneel by sitting astride some cushions. Adjust the height and padding until you are completely comfortable.

You can also sit on a chair. Make sure it has a back; an office or dining chair works best for this. Rather than leaning into the chair, it is best to sit with your lower back right up against the backrest, with your shoulders in a straight line above your hips. This will pull your upper back away from the backrest slightly, allowing you to keep your spine straight. Your legs should be uncrossed with your thighs parallel and your feet flat on the floor.

off my mobile phone and sit cross-legged on a cushion with a blanket wrapped around me. I do this regardless of whether it is hot or cold outside, as it helps me to feel comfortable and settled. When I first started meditating I was convinced I was doing it wrong. There were no fireworks, no great revelations or epiphanies; it was just me, sat on a cushion with my eyes closed. Eventually, I realized it actually is that simple. Some days my mind is racing and I feel anxious, agitated or frustrated. Other days I feel calm, centred and present. And that is the practice. No matter what state I am in, or what I experience during a meditation, I know that it is helping me in both the short and long term. It helps me to see things more clearly, to recognize my negative thought patterns, and to accept whatever arises in any given moment with more patience and compassion.

Maintaining a Regular Practice

When learning to meditate, it is important not to worry if you feel like you are doing it 'wrong' or that it is 'not working'. There is no right or wrong when it comes to meditation; only practice. As we will see in the next section, as long as you keep bringing your attention back to your breath, that is really all that matters.

Moreover, regular practice is key: all the evidence points to this being fundamental to reaping the benefits. Making time for a formal meditation, mindfulness or yoga practice is one of the most important steps you can take for your physical and mental wellbeing.

It is also worth mentioning the importance of not putting pressure on yourself. Yes, it is good to maintain a daily practice, but not at the expense of your stress levels. If you are trying to fit it in when you already feel overwhelmed or like your time is too stretched, this could actually be counterproductive. It is about finding the right balance between self-discipline and self-care. Your number-one priority should be your own wellbeing. Even if you are responsible for the wellbeing of others, you cannot care for them until you have cared for yourself first.

There is no right or wrong when it comes to meditation; only practice

USING THE BREATH IN MINDFULNESS MEDITATION

The breath is fundamental to any meditation practice. It is the one true constant, acting as an anchor and keeping you focused. This is a safe place to return your attention to again and again; it can feel like coming home.

THERE ARE MANY MEDITATIVE PRACTICES centred around the breath, from simple observing and counting techniques to more formal practices, such as the 'Mindfulness of Breathing' (page 53). It is likely that some of these practices will work better for you, or resonate more strongly with you, than others.

Personally, I have always struggled with practices involving counting the breath. I find that whenever I start to count my breath, it changes. The instructions are to simply observe the breath and to count the inhalations and exhalations in a certain way, but however simple this sounds, I usually find it quite difficult to sustain. But we know that there is no right or wrong in meditation, so I continue to practise anyway. Perhaps one day I will experience a breakthrough in breath counting. In the meantime, I prefer practices such as using an anchor for the breath (page 51) and alternate nostril breathing (page 57).

The breath is fundamental to meditation

Observing vs. Controlling the Breath

As I have found, there is a fine line between observing and controlling the breath, and it can be a challenge to simply observe it without changing it in any way. We know that awareness is key, so a good place to start with the breath is by simply observing it.

I invite you to take a moment to practise this right now. Sit comfortably with your back straight, shoulders relaxed, mouth gently closed, jaw relaxed and tongue loose. Close your eyes if you are able. Take your attention to your breath and just watch it. Try not to change it; let it be, however it is right now. Notice the qualities of it and ask yourself these questions:

- Is it shallow or deep?
- Is it fast or slow?
- Is it ragged or smooth?
- Can you feel the cool air coming in through your nose?
- Can you feel the warmer air going out through your nose?

Simply observe.

Now take a deeper, slower breath in and exhale slowly. And another. And another. How is your breath now? What changes do you notice in your body? How do you feel?

By practising this simple technique, you can begin to understand the differences between observing and controlling the breath, and perhaps you will begin to get a feel for the positive effects of working with the breath in mindful yoga.

The Breath as an Anchor

During yoga or meditation, you can return to your breath whenever you feel your attention wandering. You know the breath is your one true constant, your never-ending internal rhythm that does not falter or stray, so you can use it to 'anchor' yourself in the present moment. This can be especially helpful if you are feeling anxious, angry or panic-stricken. Taking a moment to recentre yourself can help take your mind off your problems and remind yourself that you are OK just as you are, in this very moment, right now.

Counting the Breath

In Ashtanga yoga, breath counting is an intrinsic part of the practice, and most of the asanas are held for a count of five breaths. So, once you have moved into each posture, you breathe slowly in and out five times before transitioning into the next one.

Counting the breath can be a very useful tool for keeping your mind from drifting off during meditation practice. There are many different counting techniques, from the simple to the more intricate.

One such meditation is to simply count each round of inhalation and exhalation. You can count as you inhale or as you exhale, whichever you prefer. After one full round you silently count 'one', then after the next round, 'two' and so on up to ten. If you get distracted and your mind wanders,

SIMPLE MEDITATION PRACTICE

FINDING AN ANCHOR FOR THE BREATH

1. Find a quiet place where you can sit for a few minutes without any distractions.

2. Choose a posture that feels right for you; this could be sitting on a chair, sitting cross-legged, kneeling or lying down.

3. Close your eyes and focus your mind's attention on your third eye – just behind the midpoint of your forehead.

4. As you slowly inhale through your nose, think 'Rising' as the air comes in. As you slowly exhale, still through your nose, think 'Falling' as the air goes out.

5. Notice where you feel your breath most prominently in your body. This could be on your upper lip, at the edges of your nostrils, at the back of your throat, in your chest, your diaphragm, your ribs or your belly.

6. Keep focusing your attention on this one area. This is your anchor for the breath. Imagine this area is strong and powerful and try taking a few deeper breaths to reinforce it.

7. Then let the deeper breaths go and breathe normally, still focusing on your anchor.

8. After a few more breaths, or when you are ready, gently open your eyes and come back into the room. Notice how you feel.

You might find you have a different anchor each time you practise this exercise, or you might find your anchor is always the same. Either way, you can always return to one of your anchors whenever you need to find inner calm and steadiness.

you simply return to one and start again. There is no goal; you are not trying to reach ten, and it does not matter how many times you start again at one. The point is that you are keeping your mind trained on your breath. Each time you notice you have stopped counting or lost your place, that is the crucial point of awareness; this is the core of the practice.

You can also use breath counting to control the length of your inhalation and exhalation, which can help to calm you down and make you feel more relaxed. Once you have found your comfortable position, close your eyes and take a moment to let your body settle. Then inhale slowly through your nose whilst counting up to four. Pause at the end of the inhalation, gently holding your breath, again to a slow count of four. Then slowly exhale through your nose for a count of six. Make sure the air is not allowed to suddenly escape all at once on the exhalation; instead, let it release slowly and steadily, with control. At the end of the exhalation, you can take a micro pause before inhaling for a count of four again. Repeat this for five rounds, then allow the mind and body to settle again and see how you are feeling. If you are not used to this kind of controlled breathing, it may feel a little strange at first. But with practice, it can become a very useful tool to incorporate into a daily mindful yoga practice, or whenever you feel anxious or overwhelmed.

Let it release slowly and steadily, with control

Counting also works in your mindful yoga sequence to count the number of breaths for which you hold each asana. This can help to steady your mind and standardize your practice, as you will hold most of the postures for the same breath count. Breath counting can also be useful when practising more advanced postures, as it helps to focus your mind while dealing with the challenge of the physical posture. I have found this particularly useful for the headstand, which requires a great deal of concentration and balance. Without focusing my mind on counting my breath, I would find it much harder to stay up for any length of time, as I would probably get distracted and lose my balance.

Mindfulness of Breathing

'Mindfulness of Breathing' is a core meditation practice in Theravada and Zen Buddhism and, more recently, many Western mindfulness programmes.

As the name suggests, the practice uses the breath as the focus of concentration. This simple discipline keeps your attention in the present moment, cultivating a state of mindfulness. It can be a very useful tool for counteracting anxiety and restlessness and for helping you to relax.

The mindfulness of breathing practice is divided into four stages, and spending five minutes per stage is a good way to start. I would suggest setting a timer so you can become fully absorbed in the practice.

Stage One

The first stage is very similar to the breath counting technique described above. After breathing in and out, you silently count 'one', then breathe in and out again and count 'two', and so on up to ten. If you reach ten, start again at one; if you lose count or your mind wanders, start again at one. Remember the goal is not to reach ten, but simply to keep your mind concentrated on your breath.

Stage Two

The second stage is very similar to the first, but with a subtle difference. Instead of counting at the end of the exhalation, you count just before the inhalation. Count 'one', then breathe in and out, then count 'two' and breathe in and out, and so on up to ten. This slight change means you are anticipating the next breath with your count, rather than counting after each breath has been taken.

Whenever your mind wanders, gently bring it back to the breath

Stage Three

In the third stage you drop the counting altogether. You are still aiming to keep your mind focused on your breath, but this time by simply observing it, rather than counting. Whenever your mind wanders, gently bring it back to the breath.

Stage Four

In the final stage, your focus becomes narrower. Each time you inhale and exhale, take your attention to the area around the upper lip and tip of the nose where you feel the air enter and leave your body. Try to notice the subtle sensations in this area. What does the breath feel like? Is it warm or cool? Are there any tingling or vibrating sensations? Is there anything else you notice?

Using the Breath in Mindful Yoga

The breath is fundamental to any mindful yoga practice; if you do not unify breath with movement then it is not true yoga, only physical exercise.

As with meditation, the breath acts as an anchor for your mindful yoga practice. It can help to steady you, help you go deeper into the postures, and form the underlying flow of your practice. You should never hold the breath during yoga: breathe deeply and fully whenever possible.

From my own experience, I know that it would have been much harder to practise some of the more advanced Ashtanga postures, even the easier ones, without using the breath. Generally speaking in yoga, you exhale into a posture so you can let go and relax into it, and inhale to help you come out. When you practise more challenging postures, which put

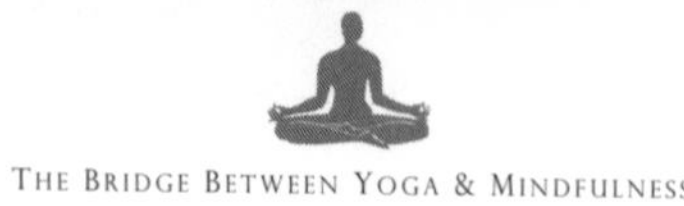

stresses and strains on certain areas of your body, your breath naturally speeds up and becomes shallower. By focusing your attention on your breath, you can use controlled awareness to start to slow it down. This will divert your mind from the physical challenge, allowing you to move more deeply and stay longer in the posture.

If you get too 'caught up' with fast, shallow breathing, this sends a message to your brain that you are in danger, that you need to panic, or that you are in 'fight or flight' mode. By encouraging your breathing to become slower and deeper, you are letting your brain know that everything is OK, you can relax, let go and feel calm.

The Relationship Between Breath & Prana

In mindful yoga we often talk about 'prana'. This is a Sanskrit word meaning 'life force' or 'life energy'. It is very similar to the Chinese *Qi* or *Chi*, which literally translates as 'breath' or 'air', but is usually interpreted as 'material energy', 'life force' or 'energy flow'. In yoga, we use the breath to control the flow of prana around the body.

What is Pranayama?

Pranayama is a practice involving breathing techniques used to balance the flow of prana within the body. 'Ayama' means 'expansion' or 'extension', so pranayama is usually interpreted as expanding, accumulating and working with prana.

MINDFUL EXERCISE

SIMPLE PRANAYAMA (YOGIC BREATHING) EXERCISE

This alternate nostril breathing exercise can help to release stress, harmonize the right and left brain hemispheres, purify the energy channels, relieve respiratory and circulatory issues, maintain body temperature and calm and centre the mind.

1. Sit in a comfortable position, either cross-legged on a mat or cushion, or on a straight-backed chair. Close your eyes.

2. Curl the index and middle finger of your right hand in towards your palm and place your right thumb on your right nostril to gently close it.

3. Slowly inhale through your left nostril only, then release your thumb and press your ring finger gently on your left nostril and breathe out slowly through your right nostril only.

4. Inhale through your right nostril, then release your ring finger and press your thumb to your right nostril and breathe out through your left nostril. This is one round.

5. Continue breathing through alternate nostrils for four more rounds, remembering to breathe in through the same nostril from which you exhaled.

6. Make sure you are breathing slowly and gently and not forcing the breath.

7. Ideally, your exhalation should be slightly longer than your inhalation. This will help you feel energized as well as relaxed.

This pranayama technique can be practised any time you feel stressed or anxious, to help with breathing problems, or to prepare the body and mind for meditation.

Pranayamic breathing exercises are often quite intricate and can be used to cleanse the body's energy channels, to bring awareness to specific areas in the body, or to generate inner heat. In Ayurveda and therapeutic yoga, pranayama is also used for recovery from illness and maintaining general health, including mood alteration and as a digestive aid. For example, *Kapalbhati Pranayama*, where you contract your stomach and make a hissing sound as you exhale, is very effective in healing stomach and digestive disorders. In fact, many people also claim it helps with weight loss.

Ujjayi Breathing

Ujjayi (pronounced oo-jye or oo-jye-ee) breath means 'victorious breath' and is often associated with yoga asana practice. It is commonly referred to as 'ocean breath' or 'oceanic breathing' because the sound produced is similar to that made by ocean waves.

The main characteristic of ujjayi breathing is a gentle restriction of the airflow in the throat, in order to control the speed and length of the breath and produce the 'rushing' ocean sound. You reduce the space at the back of your throat by gently lowering your soft palate so there is a narrower channel for the air to flow through. The sound can be likened to Darth Vader from *Star Wars* if that is more helpful! The inhalation and exhalation should be the same length and both made through the nose.

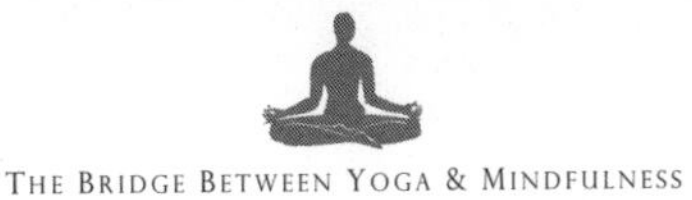

This breathing technique is encouraged throughout the asana practice of Ashtanga and other forms of yoga to help maintain a consistent rhythm throughout. Practitioners are able to stay more present, self-aware and grounded in the practice, which in turn takes on a more meditative quality. It is said that ujjayi breathing can also tone the lungs, help regulate blood pressure, build energy and internal heat, clear out toxins and encourage a free and healthy flow of prana throughout the body.

The breath is of great importance to both yoga and meditation, and therefore essential to any mindful yoga practice. In the next chapter we will explore some specific mindful practices that can be incorporated in our everyday lives, all of which include a focus on the breath at their core.

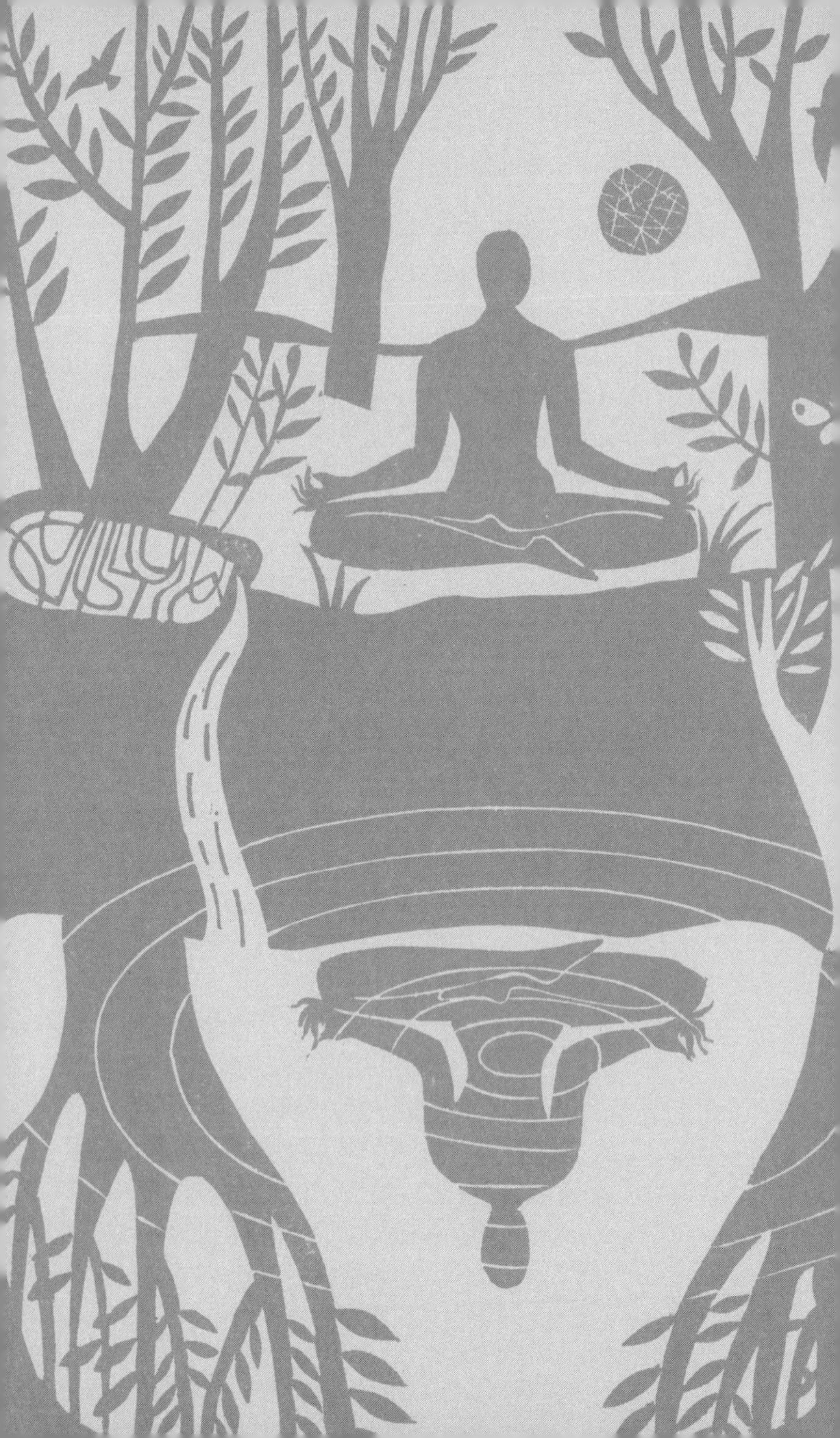

CHAPTER THREE

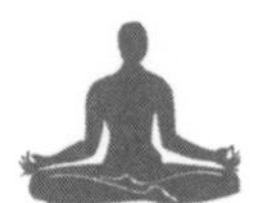

Mindful Yoga in Our Daily Lives

Stress and pressure are part of the human experience, and yogis and non-yogis alike encounter them, many on a regular basis. In small doses this can actually serve us well – it helps us get things done on a day-to-day level and can be important for survival in extreme cases, as our 'fight or flight' mode kicks in. Mindful practices can help us all to manage our stress levels to avoid them getting out of control.

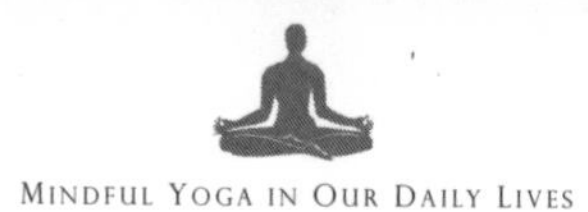

Mindfulness in the Twenty-First Century

There is no doubt that mindfulness is becoming increasingly mainstream in the West. Most people have heard of mindfulness, even if they have never practised it. It is becoming more recognized as an invaluable tool by those in positions of authority, who have responsibility for the wellbeing of others. In some countries, it is even being taught in schools and offered in prisons.

Most of us today experience the increasing pressures of modern life. We spend much of our time in busy mode: rushing around, trying to get everything done, trying to squeeze one more thing into our day. We are continuously glued to screen after screen, our attention constantly snatched away by a barrage of online information, social media feeds, smartphone notifications, data pop-ups and media attention. Our minds race and we lie awake at night, worrying about what has already passed or what might never happen.

There is a growing body of evidence (psychological, physiological and neurological) that our chaotic, stress-filled lives are causing us a great deal of damage. Many people are suffering from mental and physical health issues, the symptoms of which could be relieved by taking time out to stop, breathe and listen. Practising mindful yoga in our daily lives can be a wonderful tool for transformation.

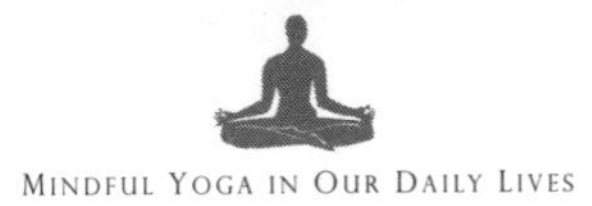

There are countless new initiatives being launched, training courses being offered and opportunities for teaching available within the realm of mindfulness. We are seeing more and more workshops and courses available to help us understand what mindfulness is and how it can help us navigate the challenges of our lives. Walk into any bookshop or library and you are bound to find at least a shelf, if not an entire section, dedicated to the topic.

All these sources recognize that mindfulness can be of huge benefit to our wellbeing. It can help to improve our concentration and mental clarity; it can help to relieve stress, anxiety, depression and chronic pain; it can affect our emotional intelligence and improve our ability to relate to ourselves and others with acceptance and kindness. It can also help us become more aware of the effects of our life choices, such as dietary decisions, time spent in front of screens and devices, how we spend our leisure time, and how we communicate and interact with others.

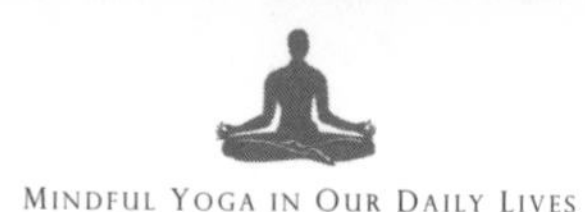

Mindfulness for Stress Relief

Feeling stressed and overwhelmed in our lives is often why we start practising in the first place. Mindfulness, meditation and yoga are all wonderful, tried-and-tested tools for tackling the effects of stress.

Spotting the Signs of Stress

Stress can come in many forms. We all know what it feels like, but sometimes it can creep up on us very gradually without us being consciously aware of it.

Feelings of worry, anxiety, pressure, panic, anger or frustration may build inside until they completely overwhelm you. You can feel utterly consumed by the feeling, as if that is all that exists in that moment: you are in a state of panic, or you become nothing but anger.

Similarly, you can get lost in repetitive thoughts, such as judging, catastrophizing, reliving, planning or rehearsing. These thoughts can become obsessive and can lead you into a negative spiral, resulting in overwhelming feelings of anxiety and, hence, you are back to feeling stressed again.

How Mindfulness Can Help

It is alarming just how quickly your brain can elevate you into a state of stress. The beauty of mindfulness is it can help you to recognize when you are getting carried away with your thoughts and stop that downward spiral from occurring.

The trick is to spot the point at which the mind has taken over and is trying to lead you into a state where you are unconsciously overwhelmed. You do this by focusing on the present moment. Catching this moment in time is the very essence of mindfulness: this is what it means to be consciously aware of this moment right now, no matter what is occurring.

The more you can train your mind to live in the present moment, the deeper your mindfulness practice will be and the lower your stress levels will become.

Standalone Mindful Practices

Before we can start practising mindful yoga, we need to take a look at mindfulness in more detail. The more we can understand its principles, the more we can start incorporating it into our daily lives, and also into our yoga practice. And the best way to do this is to learn some mindful practices.

We spend much of our time on autopilot, carrying out repetitive tasks without really noticing what we are doing. When was the last time you truly paid attention whilst you were washing the dishes or brushing your teeth? Bringing mindfulness to tasks such as these can open your eyes to a whole new perspective on life.

Consistent practice is important when it comes to mindfulness. Whichever of these mindful tools you choose to incorporate into your life, try to do so on a regular basis to maximize their benefits.

Physical Practices

Here are some activities you can try during the course of a normal day. The next time you are eating or walking, introduce a little more mindfulness and notice if you feel any differently.

Mindful Eating

In most Western cultures, eating is a very sociable activity. You might visit a restaurant for a special occasion, invite friends and family round for a meal, hold a dinner party or arrange a lunch date. Even if you are just enjoying a simple meal at home, the chances are you will be talking to other people, watching television, reading a book, or engaged in countless other activities whilst you eat.

This means your attention is not wholly focused on eating. But what would happen if it was? There is a Zen Buddhist saying that goes, 'When walking, just walk'. In other words, focus your attention on one simple activity at a time. This can be applied to other activities too: 'When cooking, just cook', 'When brushing your teeth, just brush your teeth', 'When eating, just eat'. So, what if you tried focusing all your attention on the activity of eating and nothing else?

One of the ways to help you do this is by counting your chews. It is claimed that chewing each mouthful of food

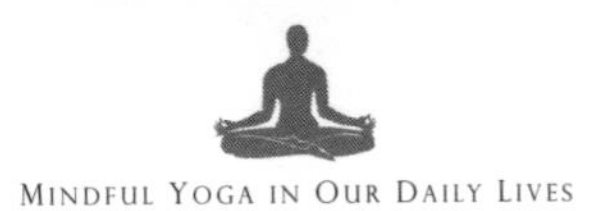

thirty to forty times can have huge benefits for both your digestive system and your state of mind. As a large proportion of the digestive process actually happens in the mouth, with your saliva breaking down the food particles, it makes sense that you should chew as many times as possible to avoid swallowing large chunks of food that your stomach will find harder to process.

Counting like this keeps your mind focused on the act of eating, and therefore forces you to stay in the present moment. You can also bring your senses into play as you notice and explore the different shapes, textures and tastes of the food in your mouth. Whenever you can, I would encourage you to try eating mindfully. It is best practised alone, or in silence, when you can be free from any distractions. Try closing your eyes and focusing only on the food as it enters and moves around your mouth. You might find you never experience eating in quite the same way again!

When walking, just walk. When eating, just eat.

Mindful Walking

If you tend to walk a lot, the chances are you spend much of the time walking the same routes. You might take the same way to work every day, go the same route into town, or have a favourite path you follow for fitness or leisure. When

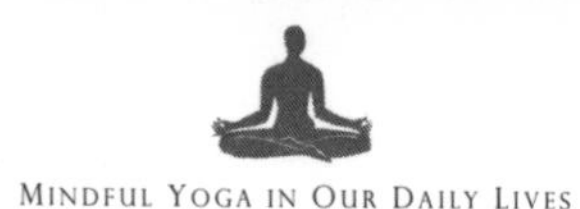

walking these familiar tracks, how often have you looked around you and truly taken in your surroundings? How often have you looked up at the buildings and trees? Or really studied the views and landscapes you can see?

The practice of mindful walking can open your eyes and allow you to see things you might never have noticed before. It also tends to slow you down, so it can be a useful tool if you often walk very fast or rush from one place to the next. See if you can leave just five or ten minutes earlier and take time to really notice what is around you the next time you are walking a familiar route.

Mental Practices

These next two practices involve communication with other people; try them out next time you find yourself engaged in a meaningful conversation, particularly with a loved one, or someone you have difficulty with.

Loving Speech

The practice of loving speech is something that can develop over a lifetime, but you might want to make a concerted effort to manifest it in your life right now. The main principle of loving speech is taking the time to think before you speak. Our words can cause much joy and happiness in others, as well as pain, doubt, frustration or anger. We often do not realize the power our words can have on others.

Loving speech includes speaking the truth, as well as avoiding the use of bad, coarse or offensive language. You can also try to bring more kindness and compassion into your words. Before you speak you might ask yourself questions, such as:

- Is it true?
- Is it kind?
- Is it helpful?
- Is it timely?

Occasionally, it might be kinder not to tell someone the whole truth, or to hold some information back. It really depends on the situation, which is why it is important to ask, 'Is it kind?' as well as, 'Is it true?' Similarly, it might not be the right time to utter certain words, or it might be kinder to speak them at a later date or in a different situation.

Pausing before you speak to ask yourself these questions, and to consider how your words might affect the listener, is a very mindful practice that can have a huge impact on your relationships and the way you interact with others.

Deep Listening

Deep listening is a practice that I believe could have benefits for us all: if every person were able to do this in each of their interactions with others, the world would be a much more harmonious place.

How often have you found yourself listening to another's words whilst simultaneously planning what to say next? Or

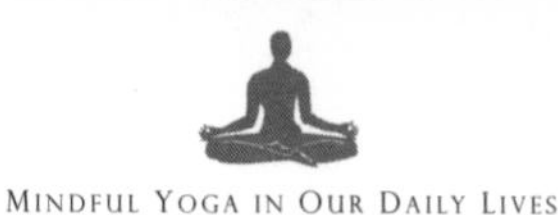

trying to think of some helpful piece of advice to give them? Or feeling the need to share a similar experience you have had in an effort to reassure them? We all do this. In fact, I would go so far as to say we all do this most of the time. It is human nature. But the problem is, if you are experiencing any of these thoughts while someone else is talking to you, then you are not fully listening to the words they are saying: you are multitasking.

The other person might have come to you to share an experience or problem, feeling a certain vulnerability and a need to be heard. If you instead give them advice, offer counselling or share your own personal stories, the chances are they will be left feeling unheard and misunderstood. As Marshall B. Rosenberg, author of *Nonviolent Communication: A Language of Life*, so eloquently puts it, 'Believing we have to "fix" situations and make others feel better prevents us from being present.'

Sure, there might be times when the other person genuinely wants your advice and even asks for it. They might be very interested to hear your own experiences, or they might want you to console them and offer your sympathy. But, there will be other times – and I am willing to bet these are in the majority – when the other person simply wants to feel heard.

So what would happen if you dropped the multitasking and just focused on a single activity: listening? You might find you hear their words slightly differently. You might find you understand them a little better. You might notice subtle cues about their underlying feelings. You might even get a sense of the unspoken needs hidden beneath their words. For we all have unspoken needs hidden beneath our words, at least some of the time, when we are talking to others.

In mindfulness we call this 'deep listening'. This means allowing yourself to be completely present with the other person and to listen with your whole being. Once you have fully heard and absorbed their words and you are sure they are ready for you to speak, only then offer words of your own, based on an authentic and intuitive response. It also means practising asking for permission before offering advice or reassurance to the other. This might feel a little strange at first, but the more you do it, the easier it becomes. I definitely have not nailed this one myself yet, but there are friends I can bring to mind who have. And when they ask if I mind them interjecting or offering their opinion, I actually feel more valued and heard, and have more respect for them in the process.

Breathe deeply, put down your own agenda and listen with your whole being

Loving speech and deep listening often go hand in hand. When you are the one talking and you feel like the other person is not fully listening, you can use loving speech to communicate your needs to them. You might politely ask

MINDFUL EXERCISE

HOW TO PRACTISE DEEP LISTENING

Try practicisng this whenever you find yourself listening to another's words. This could be in a casual, social setting, or a more formal, professional one. It can be particularly useful if someone is confiding in you, sharing sensitive information or dealing with a challenging situation.

1. Keep your attention focused on the person and try not to get distracted by other noises or movement around you. If you find that you do get distracted, just keep bringing your attention back to the person's words.

2. Breathe deeply, put down your own agenda and listen with your whole being.

3. As thoughts and judgements arise (which they will), try not to engage with them; simply observe them and let them go again.

4. When you feel the need to interject (which you undoubtedly will), remind yourself that it is not necessary. Think of this time as sacred for the other person; it is their moment to speak and yours will come soon.

5. The keys here are empathy and compassion. The more deeply you are able to listen to the other person, the more empathy and compassion you are likely to feel for them, and the more of these you feel, the more likely you are to continue listening deeply.

6. When the person's speech reaches a natural pause, this is your turn to talk. You might need to take a moment to collect your thoughts, and you can even let them know this if it feels appropriate. Before you speak, remember to ask yourself, 'Is it true? Is it kind? Is it helpful? Is it timely?'

them not to interrupt, or gently explain that you are not looking for advice and simply need to feel heard. Again, this might take some getting used to, but I believe the clearer we can be in our communications, the better for all involved.

Loving Kindness

Practising loving kindness is a wonderful way to evoke feelings of compassion and empathy, towards both yourself and others. Similar to the mindful practices, loving kindness can be incorporated into your mindful yoga or meditation practice; however, it warrants its own section here, as it is a comprehensive meditation with several different layers and versions.

Loving kindness meditation comes from the Theravadan Buddhist tradition and is also known as *Metta Bhavana* or 'metta meditation'. The word *metta* comes from the Pali language (in Sanskrit *maitri)* and means 'loving kindness' or 'goodwill'. It is about cultivating a sense of kindness and compassion towards all living beings, including yourself.

There are many different ways to practise loving kindness, and I have included three versions here which I have personally found useful. They all share the same basic principle of reciting a mantra whilst focusing your attention on a different person or group of people. The mantra usually has four lines, but again they vary widely, depending on which source you follow.

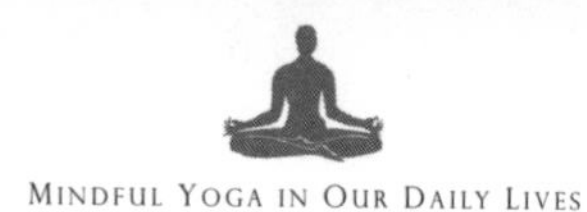

Here are some of the more common lines that can be included in your mantra:

May I be happy just as I am.

May I be healthy and strong.

May I be safe and free from harm.

May I be peaceful and at ease.

May I be free from all suffering.

May I be able to live joyously and with love.

May my life be filled with happiness, health and wellbeing.

It is important that the words you recite in your mantra carry meaning for you and are easy to remember. I suggest you experiment with different versions and choose the one that most resonates with you. For the examples that follow, I shall use this version:

May I be happy.

May I be healthy.

May I be free from all suffering.

May I be peaceful and at ease.

To incorporate loving kindness into your yoga practice, try applying each stage of the technique to a particular posture, or set of postures. You can recite your mantra whilst holding each posture, breathing deeply as you silently repeat each line in your head. I find standing postures work well for this, particularly the stronger standing poses such as Warrior (*Virabhadrasana*), Triangle (*Trikonasana*) and Side Angle Pose (*Utthita Parsvakonasana*).

Loving Kindness: Version One

This is probably the most common version of the Metta Bhavana and involves sending loving kindness first to yourself, then to a loved one, then to a neutral person, and lastly to someone you have difficulty with.

Sending Loving Kindness to Yourself

Start by finding a comfortable position, either sitting on a chair, sitting or kneeling on a cushion, or lying down. Close your eyes and take a few deep breaths in and out through your nose. Then continue to breathe gently and naturally.

Now, repeat your mantra several times, either silently or out loud:

May I be happy.
May I be healthy.
May I be free from all suffering.
May I be peaceful and at ease.

This meditation is all about feeling good, so it is important that you feel comfortable. Try to 'drop' into your heart space by taking your attention to the area around your heart and focusing on feelings of pure love and empathy that emanate from there. If negative feelings, such as judgement, criticism or hatred arise – either for yourself or others – try to gently let them go again and come back to your breath. Focus on softening and opening your heart space, by allowing feelings of acceptance and compassion to arise.

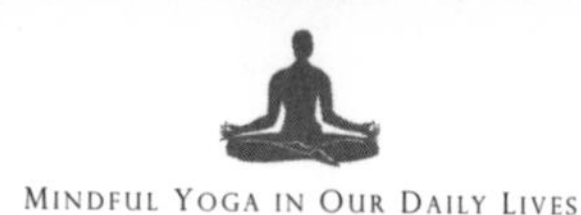

Sending Loving Kindness to a Loved One

Next, bring to mind a loved one – someone for whom you feel a great fondness, or who evokes a feeling of pure, unconditional love. This could be a partner, family member, close friend or even a pet. With the same opening and softening from your heart, focus your attention on this being and send them your compassion and goodwill. It can be helpful to visualize them standing in front of you, receiving your loving kindness whilst you repeat your mantra to them:

May you be happy.
May you be healthy.
May you be free from all suffering.
May you be peaceful and at ease.

Sending Loving Kindness to a Neutral Person

For the third stage, bring to mind a neutral person, someone for whom you have no strong feelings either way. This is usually someone you have met but do not know very well. They could be an acquaintance, a colleague, a familiar shopkeeper or a neighbour you say hello to every day.

Repeat your mantra, allowing yourself to feel tenderness towards this person. Even though you might not know or understand very much about them, you can still send them loving kindness and concern for their welfare. Try to visualize this person in the context in which you usually see them, and imagine smiling kindly at them as you recite your mantra.

Sending Loving Kindness to Someone You Have Difficulty With

Lastly, bring to mind someone you have difficulty with. This could be someone you dislike, someone with whom you are in conflict, or someone you feel resentment or hostile feelings towards.

This is the stage that many people find the hardest, as it can feel uncomfortable focusing on conflict or ill-feeling towards others. Try to reconnect with the positive feelings you have towards your loved ones. If you find it too challenging to visualize this person standing in front of you and repeating your mantra to them, you can distance yourself slightly by reciting it in the third person:

May [name] be happy.
May [name] be healthy.
May [name] be free from all suffering.
May [name] be peaceful and at ease.

Loving Kindness: Version Two

In this second version, you begin by sending loving kindness to yourself in exactly the same way as before.

Then you gradually widen the circle of your focus to larger groups of people, starting with your immediate surroundings. So, you might send loving kindness to all beings within the room, building or community that you are currently in. Recite your mantra several times, focusing your attention on the people in this area. Then you can widen this to all beings

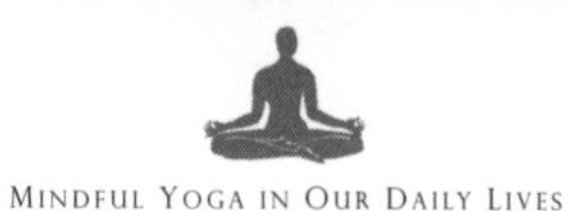

within the town, city or country, and finally to all beings on the planet:

May all beings be happy.

May all beings be healthy.

May all beings be free from all suffering.

May all beings be peaceful and at ease.

Loving Kindness: Version Three

The first two versions rely on being able to send loving kindness to yourself first, before focusing on others. This is good practice, as you need to be able to cultivate feelings of love and compassion for yourself before you can start cultivating these feelings for others.

However, in Western cultures in particular, many people find it difficult to send loving feelings towards themselves. They may feel selfish or self-indulgent, unworthy or undeserving of happiness when others are suffering. In these cases, it may be helpful to practise this third version, at least to begin with.

In version three, you start where it is easiest – sending loving kindness to your loved ones. Then, as you open your heart little by little, you can start directing these feelings to areas where you find it more difficult.

Bring to mind someone who loves you very much and send your loving kindness to them whilst repeating your mantra, as you did in version one. Then, repeat this with another person

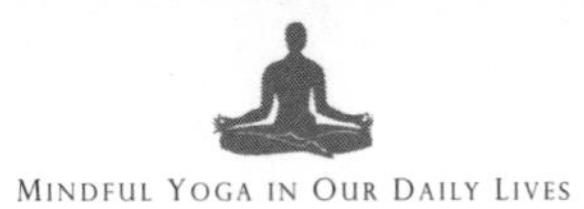

you deeply love and care about. These people can be from the past or present.

Next, visualize these two people standing or sitting either side of you as they offer you their loving kindness in return. Imagine the expressions on their faces and their body language as they both recite the mantra to you:

May you be happy.

May you be healthy.

May you be free from all suffering.

May you be peaceful and at ease.

You may find it helpful to place your hand on your heart or imagine yourself bathed in a warm, golden light, as you receive their love and good wishes. If you struggle to send loving kindness to yourself, you should find this version helps, by imagining people dear to you sending you their loving kindness instead.

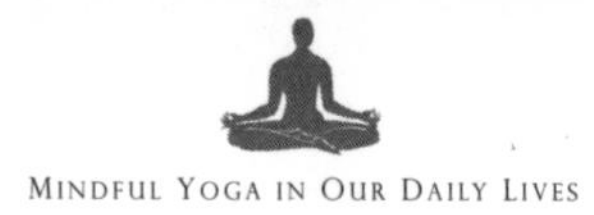

Mindful Practices for Yoga or Meditation

The practices in this section can be used as standalone tools, but also work well when incorporated into your mindful yoga or mindfulness meditation practice.

Yoga is much more than just a physical practice. Once you start incorporating it into your life, it can start to affect your values, ethical principles and relationships, as well as your general outlook on life. Just like mindfulness, it has the power to change everything. We know that yoga goes far beyond merely asana practice, therefore the more mindful our yoga practice can become, the more mindful our lives can potentially become.

Body Scan

Sometimes, merely focusing on your breath is not enough to take you out of your repetitive thoughts and into the present moment, and you need a stronger distraction from your overwhelmed mind. In cases such as these, you might find a body scan more helpful.

You can practise the body scan whilst seated in a chair, on a cushion, or even lying down on your back. Many people prefer to lie down, as it helps you to fully relax and let your body sink into the floor. For this reason, it is the perfect

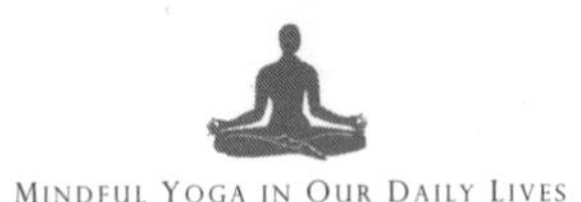

meditation for Corpse Pose (*Shavasana*) at the end of your yoga practice. You can take anywhere from five to twenty minutes to complete this exercise, depending on the time you have available.

Close your eyes and take three deep breaths to relax into your body. Then, starting at the top of your head, focus on each area of your body at a time, bringing your awareness to it and encouraging it to relax. You do not need to physically move that part of your body; simply bringing your awareness to it and imagining the release of tension is enough.

You might want to give yourself a running commentary in your head, as if someone else was guiding the body scan. So, you might say to yourself, 'Bring your awareness to the top of your head, the sides of your head, the back of your head. Relax your forehead, relax around your eyes, your cheeks and your nose. Allow your tongue to drop to the back of your mouth, with your lips gently touching and your jaw relaxed. Be aware of the back of the neck and the throat, relax the tops of the shoulders,' and so on.

If you find it easier, you can listen to a guided body scan meditation. There are many audio files available, via MP3s, apps, streaming services or CDs. Whichever method you choose, make sure you place your attention completely on each body part as you slowly scan through your body. This will ensure that your mind is fully in the present moment and far less likely to get distracted by your thoughts.

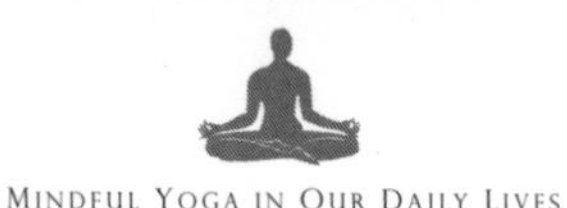

Focusing on Sounds

Another tool that many people find helpful to bring them into the present moment is focusing on sounds. You can do this either as a structured meditation or just by taking a moment to stop whatever you happen to be doing. It also works well as a seated meditation as part of your yoga practice, or whilst lying in Corpse Pose (Shavasana) at the end.

Close your eyes and take three deep breaths to fully 'arrive' in this moment. Focus on the air as it travels in through your nose, down the back of your throat, into your lungs, past your ribcage and down into your stomach. Now, listen carefully to your surroundings and notice what you can hear. There might be sounds close by or far away, loud or quiet, short and sharp or continuous drones.

If you are indoors, you might be able to hear someone in the next room, or a neighbour in the next building. Perhaps your refrigerator is humming or your mobile phone sends an alert. Outside, you might be able to hear birds singing or traffic driving past, perhaps people's voices or a sudden bang.

Whatever sounds you hear, try not to attach any meaning or judgement to them. You are simply a curious observer taking in all that you hear. Try not to fixate on any one sound, but keep your ears open for whatever might arise next. By focusing your attention purely on the sounds you can hear, you are keeping your mind attuned to what is happening in real time in this very moment, right now.

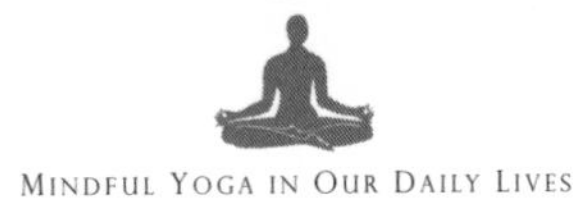

Labelling Thoughts

Labelling thoughts is a useful practice for distancing yourself from the constant chatter of your mind. It can be particularly beneficial if you spend a lot of time getting lost in your thoughts, finding your mind going off on tangents and feeling overwhelmed by your thought processes, especially when this leads to negative thoughts spiralling out of control.

You can use this technique during a formal yoga or meditation practice, or simply throughout the day whenever the moment arises. The most important – and most challenging – part of this practice is to 'catch' the moment when you realize you have become lost in your thoughts. If you are practising yoga or meditation, then this is the point at which you realize your mind is no longer focused on your breath, or on the synchronicity between your breath and your movement. If you are applying this practice to the course of your normal day, then this is the point when you start to feel overwhelmed by your thoughts, or you realize your thoughts have become repetitive or obsessive.

Once you have caught the moment, you can then apply a label to your thoughts. You might realize you were caught up in planning-type thoughts, such as wondering what to have for dinner, or considering a difficult discussion with a colleague. You might have been dwelling on some aspect of the past, such as wishing you had done something differently, or going over a previous conversation in your head. There are

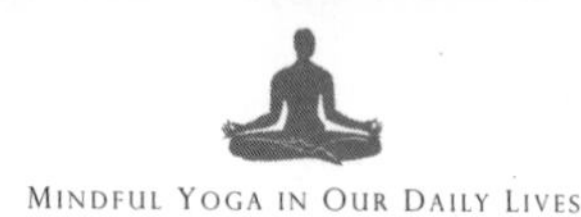

many types of thoughts that can become obsessive and spiral out of control; here are a few of the most common:

- Planning
- Criticizing
- Rehearsing
- Reliving
- Regressing
- Worrying
- Obsessing
- Catastrophizing

You might want to come up with your own labels as you become more familiar with this practice. Catching the moments when you have become lost in your thoughts and applying labels to them should help you to distance yourself from them. The more you can separate yourself from your thoughts, the more you will be able to see them as just that – thoughts. And thoughts are not necessarily real. In time, it will become clearer which of your thoughts are helpful to you and which ones you can simply observe, label as unhelpful and let go again.

Gratitude Practice

Practising gratitude is a wonderful way of bringing more positivity into your life. Rather than focusing on what you do not have, or on what is missing from your life, gratitude helps you to focus on what you do have and express appreciation for it.

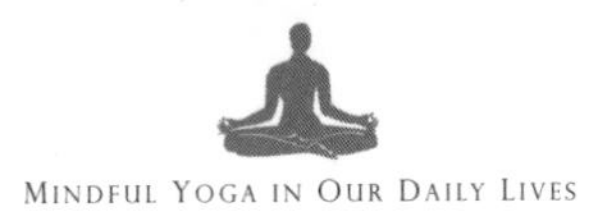

Everyone has things for which they can be grateful, even if you might not think so at first. If you can develop a regular gratitude practice, you will become more mindful of all the positive things in your life, which can be self-perpetuating – the more gratitude you feel, the happier you will become; the happier you become, the more gratitude you will feel. This can be a very useful tool in helping to manage symptoms of unhappiness, anxiety and depression.

Focus on what you do have and express appreciation for it

Gratitude is a wonderful tool to incorporate into yoga. Whilst sitting in meditation at the beginning of your practice, or lying in Corpse Pose (Shavasana) at the end, with each breath you can breathe in gratitude and breathe out love. If it helps, you can visualize your whole body being filled with a bright, golden light as you breathe in gratitude to every part of your body. You can then visualize sending this light out to all living beings as you breathe out.

You can also bring gratitude into the actual asanas. For each posture you move into, choose something in your life you feel grateful for. As you hold the posture, breathing deeply and steadily, focus on the feeling of gratitude as you think about that aspect of your life. You can choose a different aspect for each posture or set of postures. This practice is particularly suited to strong standing poses such as Warrior

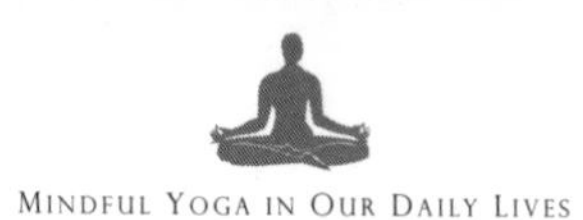

MINDFUL EXERCISE

KEEPING A GRATITUDE JOURNAL

Simple Version

1. Before you go to sleep, think about what happened during that day: where you went, who you saw, what you did, how you felt.

2. Write down three things you feel grateful for. These could be related to that specific day, for example, 'I am grateful I got to the meeting on time', or, 'I am grateful for my partner's support in dealing with this problem'. Or, they could relate to your life in general, for example, 'I am grateful that I have a loving family around me', or, 'I am grateful for the financial stability my job provides me'.

3. Do not do this exercise on autopilot; really think about the positive aspects of your life and notice how they make you feel.

4. Try to incorporate this exercise into your daily routine, but try to release any pressure around it. The more of an obligation this practice becomes, the more your autopilot will kick in, meaning it will not be coming from an authentic place.

Extended Version

5. As well as listing three things you are grateful for each day, you can also include:

a two unexpected things that happened that day; and

b two people you are grateful for.

6. As you wake up, list three things that would brighten your day. This should kick-start your morning by creating a more positive frame of mind. The trick here is not to put pressure on yourself to actually make these things happen. Having the positive thoughts in the first place is the most important part of this practice.

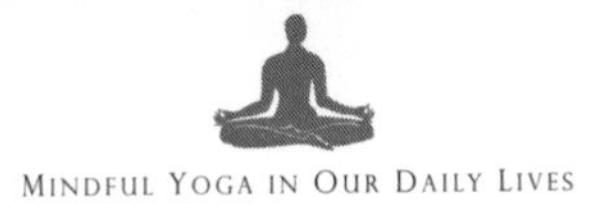

(Virabhadrasana), Triangle (Trikonasana) and Side Angle Pose (Utthita Parsvakonasana).

A good way to get into the habit of practising gratitude is to write gratitude lists or, better yet, to keep a gratitude journal. You can make these lists in your head, before you go to bed or as you wake up. I would recommend writing in a journal at the end of the day, as this allows for reflection on the day's activities and works as a reminder of all you have to be grateful for.

Hopefully you are now equipped with plenty of tools for incorporating more mindfulness into your day-to-day life. It might feel overwhelming at first, so I would encourage you to start small. Pick one or two practices that you like the sound of and see if you can start bringing them in at relevant opportunities. For example, you could try focusing on sounds next time you are washing the dishes, mindful eating next time you are dining alone, or thinking of three things you are grateful for each night for a week before you go to bed. In the final chapter we will see how we can incorporate some of these practices into a mindful yoga sequence.

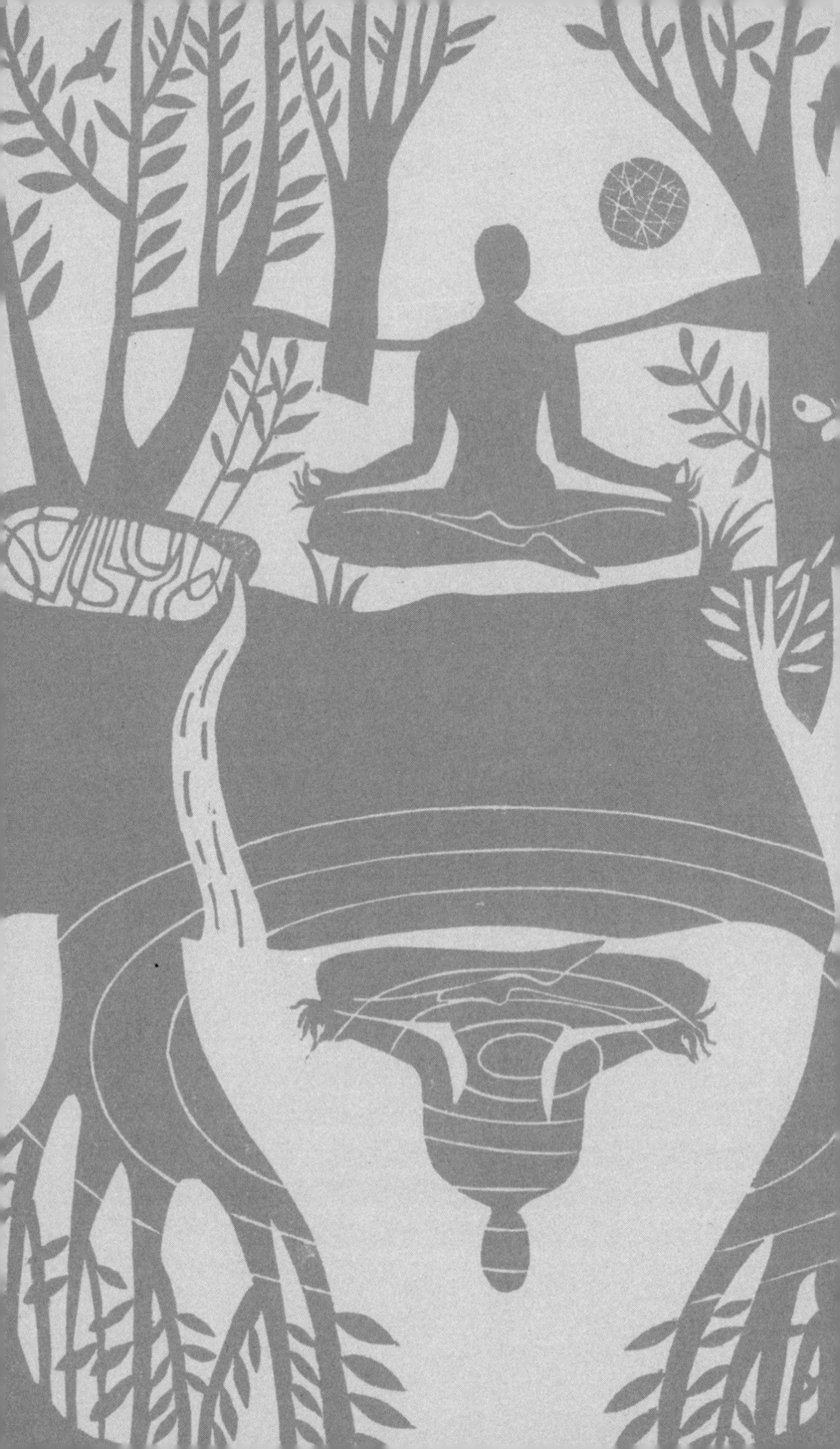

CHAPTER FOUR

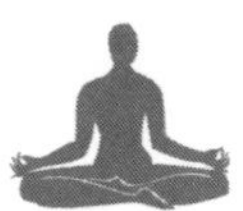

Mindful Yoga in the Twenty-First Century

Our perception of yoga in the West has changed drastically over the last ten years. It has become increasingly mainstream and is now big business in many countries. Everyone, it seems, wants to be a yoga teacher, so what part do teachers and teacher training play in the changing face of modern yoga? What are some of the risks of practising yoga without mindfulness at its heart? And how can you find your way on the right path in this confusing landscape?

The Changing Face of Modern Yoga

In recent years, particularly in the West, we have seen a huge increase in the popularity of yoga. But is yoga developing into something far removed from its Eastern origins?

When I first discovered yoga, it was practised by a minority of people, the kind of activity you would find on the noticeboards of local halls and venues. It had an air of mystique around it and was primarily seen as an Eastern or spiritual practice.

Today, the yoga landscape looks very different. Every major city has at least one yoga studio, if not a plethora. Most gyms and fitness studios offer some form of yoga on their timetable. Wherever you live, it seems you do not have to go far to find a class. And most locations now offer a wide choice of different styles and teachers from a variety of different traditions.

Yoga classes, workshops and private tuition are available for pregnant women, mothers with newborn babies, toddlers, teenagers, the over-fifties and men only. You can find classes in yoga therapy, yoga for anxiety and depression, yoga for back pain and yoga for weight loss. All sorts of weird and wonderful fads are being developed around the world all the time. You can now experience such delights as naked yoga, yoga raves, beer yoga, doga (yoga with dogs), goat yoga, paddleboard yoga, rage yoga, cannabis yoga and even Harry Potter yoga!

The more serious yoga classes are changing too. Classical yoga started as a very spontaneous and intuitive practice, then developed into a set of static, standardized poses as its popularity grew. Recently, we have seen the introduction of more flowing sequences, which are sometimes described as dance-like, and often set to music. And with the modern mindfulness movement, we are now seeing a return to a more authentic style, as we look at ways to introduce more awareness and presence into our yoga practice.

Yoga in the Digital Age

The rise of the internet, social media and smartphones has led to total euphoria for the digital yogi. You do not have to look far online to find the latest yoga blog, yoga podcast, online yoga course or digital yoga products. If you indicate yoga-related interests in your social media profiles, then your Facebook news feed is likely to be crammed full of the latest 'how-to' videos from advanced practitioners and teachers. Yoga media figures and celebrities have completely altered the public perception of the practice. For many, yoga has become a fashion statement.

The truth is, many of us want that feel-good factor. And we want it now. In our increasingly fast-paced world, we expect instant results. We gain much of our self-worth through comparison with others. So perhaps we feel the need to tweet about our recent 'accomplishment' of an advanced pose, or blog about the life-changing experience we had on a yoga retreat.

This all begs the question, 'Do you need to be posting your latest yoga selfies on social media, and publishing your green smoothie of the month on your yoga blog, in order to be a good yoga student or teacher in the modern world?' My answer to this question is, 'No you don't, unless it feels right for you.' As long as what you are doing, and the way you behave online, is in keeping with your own values and beliefs, then go for it! However, if you are jumping on the 'yoga bandwagon' just for the sake of it, because you feel you 'should', or because you feel pressured to, then I would argue that you are not practising yoga mindfully.

Yoga is Big Business

Aside from the actual classes, workshops and one-to-one tuition available, it seems there is a lot of money to be made in the yoga industry. Yoga retreats and holidays are becoming more and more popular as people increasingly desire to feel nourished and energized, in contrast to their busy, stressful lives. Yoga 'superstars' and almost-celebrity teachers charge high prices for their world tours, attracting students from far and wide.

Visit any bookshop or library and you will find a seemingly endless supply of information on yoga: its history, philosophy, different traditions, different styles, practice manuals, study references and personal accounts. Pick up any yoga magazine, or do a quick search online, and you will find countless businesses offering yoga clothes, equipment and accessories.

We are constantly trying to better ourselves: to become slimmer, stronger, kinder, happier, more likeable. We want to believe what we hear in the media, or from our peers and colleagues. We follow fashion and weight-loss trends so that we can become better connected and feel a sense of belonging. So, we try the latest yoga fad and make sure we own a pair of the latest yoga leggings.

The most important question to ask ourselves is, 'How does it feel on the inside?'

Yoga, without a doubt, is booming in the West, and this is a trend that is surely set to increase. The most important question to ask ourselves when searching for that yoga 'fix', however, is not about how it looks from the outside, but, 'How does it feel on the inside?'

MINDFUL YOGA EXERCISE

YOGA ASANA: DOWNWARD DOG (ADHO MUKHA SVANASANA)

This is a very simple yet effective yoga asana. If you only have time to practise one posture a day, make it this one!

1. Start by coming on to 'all fours' on your mat with your shoulders above your wrists and your hips above your knees.

2. Inhale, curl your toes under, then exhale, lift your knees off the mat, straighten your legs and push your hips up towards the ceiling to come into an upside down 'V' position.

3. Keep your fingers spread evenly and your palms pressed into the mat. Relax your shoulders down, away from your ears.

4. Take a few deep breaths, focusing your attention on the air as it travels in and out through your body. Do not try to change the breath; simply observe it.

5. If you feel like moving, move. Try bending one knee at a time to stretch and release the hamstrings, or lift one leg off the floor at a time, stretching it up and back.

6. Your heels might not reach the ground to begin with (or ever) and this is perfectly fine. It's more important to keep pushing up and back through the shoulders and hips to stretch the arms and legs.

7. Now, take your attention to different areas of your body. There might be areas that feel tense or tight. Can you use your breath to breathe into these areas and soften the tension?

8. The most important thing is to tune in to your body. How is it feeling? What does it need right now? Does this feel good? How about this? Be curious. Be playful. Be mindful.

9. When finished, drop your knees to the floor and rest on your mat.

The Role of the Teacher in Mindful Yoga

The yoga teacher's role is of critical importance. Their attitude, the words they use to describe the practice, the thoughts and feelings they evoke in you, the way they adjust you in the asanas, the inspiration or encouragement they develop in you – all of these have a bearing on your personal approach to the practice.

My first yoga teacher was a gentle soul. She had a kind smile and a soft voice. I felt safe and supported by her. When she taught a class, she held the space calmly and confidently. I could tell she was passionate about the practice and that it had helped her in her life. I felt inspired by her and wanted to experience some of the inner joy, contentment and peace that she clearly exuded.

I have practised yoga with many teachers since then and one thing that has stood out – that has drawn me closer to some in particular – is their journey. The teachers I have found most inspirational are those who have clearly been through the process themselves. They have experienced some form of struggle in their life – be it mild or significant, mental or physical, emotional or psychological – and they have turned to yoga to help them. They are clearly passionate about the practice and want to share it with others, encouraging healing and transformation wherever it is needed.

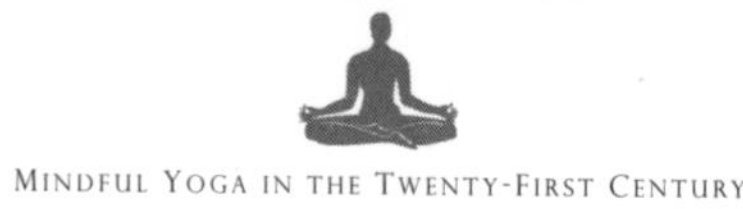

At the same time, though, these teachers are not preachers or activists. They do not try to force yoga on everyone, or assume that others will have the same experience they had. They are simply sharing their knowledge and wisdom in the hopes that others will benefit from the effects of the practice, as they have.

I believe a good yoga teacher should guide a student's practice, not dictate it. They should know when to push and encourage and when to step back and simply observe. Ideally, they will have the opportunity to get to know their students individually, so that they can help to shape each student's practice in the most effective way for them. In a conference in Mysore in March 2014, R. Sharath Jois expressed this perfectly, using the analogy of a coconut tree. He explained that your teacher can show you where the coconut tree is and give you some tips on how to climb it, but ultimately you have to climb the tree yourself.

Can One Size Fit All?

I think one of the issues facing many teacher training programmes – and indeed many styles of yoga – today, is that they subscribe to the 'one size fits all' approach. There is too much emphasis on achieving the perfect posture. Most teachers talk of 'modifications' or 'variations' of an asana, in case you are unable to bend yourself into its full state. I do think it is useful to know the full state of each asana, but perhaps the language we use to describe this could be altered to allow more inclusivity and less negativity.

For example, teachers in mindful yoga classes I have attended give instructions such as, 'Now bend forwards from the hips as far as is comfortable for you. You might come to here or you might come to here; it does not matter; what matters is that you keep your chest lifted and your spine lengthened.' To me, this is the sign of a good teacher: talking about how the posture feels, rather than how it looks.

As human beings we are fascinatingly similar, yet wonderfully unique. We come in all shapes and sizes, in varying proportions and with different levels of strength and flexibility. So, if one person can put their hands flat on the floor in a standing forward bend, whereas another is a long way from reaching their toes, it really does not matter; they are still practising yoga, and they will still reap the rewards from the practice. It is only our egos that tell us otherwise.

Following on from this is the debate around using props in your yoga practice. Some people disapprove, but I believe props are an invaluable part of mindful yoga, as they add extra height, length or support where needed. For example, when sitting cross-legged, many people tend to slouch their shoulders, and sitting on a block can help to alleviate this, by encouraging the spine to come into a more upright position. If you cannot reach your toes in a seated forward bend, looping a belt around your feet and gradually moving your

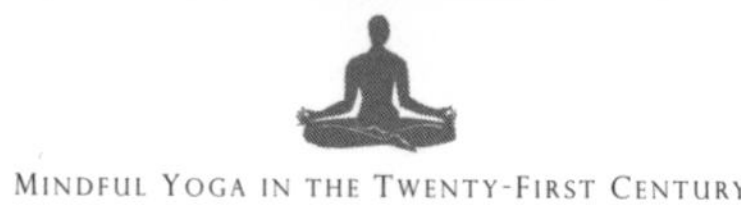

hands down the belt can help you to mindfully release more deeply into the posture without assistance.

I would argue that when it comes to yoga, one size cannot possibly fit all. Not everyone will be attracted to yoga and not everyone will experience the same effects from the practice. Certain styles will resonate differently with different people. Some students will feel inspired and supported by a certain teacher; others will feel an aversion to them. The most important thing is to find what works for you.

THE RISKS OF MINDLESS YOGA

We have looked at why mindfulness is so important in yoga, and some ways to bring more mindfulness into our practice. But, what happens when we do not do this? What are some of the risks associated with practising yoga less mindfully?

OVER THE LAST TWENTY YEARS OR SO, I have practised yoga in many different ways, with countless teachers, in numerous locations, and I have witnessed thousands of fellow practitioners doing the same. I have seen some of the negative aspects of yoga, the difficulties and challenges many people – including myself – have faced. I firmly believe that many of these issues – particularly the more physical ones – were caused by practitioners engaging in the opposite of mindful yoga: mindless yoga.

My Sore Knee

There is a long-standing joke amongst Ashtanga practitioners to refer to Mysore in India, the birthplace of Ashtanga yoga, as 'My sore knee', or 'My sore back' and so on. Particularly for those outside the Ashtanga community (aside only from Bikram or hot yoga), it has a reputation as being the most dynamic, the most intense, and therefore the most injury-prone of all the yoga styles.

There is a difference between 'good' pain and 'bad' pain

During the six months I spent in Mysore, not a day would pass without at least one fellow practitioner discussing or complaining about their latest injury. From torn menisci in the knees and rotator cuff injuries in the shoulders, to pulled hamstrings and severe lower back pain, it seemed almost everyone was suffering from a yoga-related affliction.

Of course, a certain amount of pain can be a good thing: 'No pain, no gain.' But there is a difference between 'good' pain and 'bad' pain. Good pain is when you can feel your muscles working. It might be a strong sensation and it might feel uncomfortable, but you can use the breath to relax through the pain. And when you tune into your body, you know it is doing you good; you know your muscles need this stretch. Bad pain, however, can be more sudden, like a sharp, shooting sensation. This is your body's way of telling you to stop. Your muscles, your joints, your brain are all saying, 'No'. As a yoga practitioner – indeed, when working with the body in any way – it is very important to know the difference.

I believe that the majority of yoga-induced injuries could be avoided using mindfulness. Perhaps you have pushed yourself just a little bit too hard; perhaps you kept ignoring a strong niggle that kept getting worse; perhaps you allowed a teacher to adjust you in a posture even though it did not feel right. Our egos can be a very powerful force when we are trying to do better, go further, become stronger or last longer, or when we are trying to impress our teachers and fellow practitioners. If, however, you are able to truly listen to your own body, trust your intuition and block out the egotistical thoughts – comparing yourself to others and worrying what other people think – you will only do what is right for you, which makes injury far less likely to occur.

Following the Herd

When we constantly turn our attention outward – towards our teacher's instructions, other practitioners' achievements, or trends in the press or social media – we are not being mindful. We need to strike a balance between acceptance of the outside world, and awareness of our inner landscape.

There was a time when, as an Ashtanga practitioner, I wanted to be a 'good' student – so I took very literally the guidelines for yoga practice, the dietary regulations and the behavioural and lifestyle rules to follow in order to be a 'good yogi'. However, my guru was living in a very different culture to me, with a very different background, upbringing and daily experience of life. So of course, I found it very difficult to apply his guidelines to my own life, resulting in those familiar feelings of pressure, inadequacy and, ultimately, failure.

In mindful yoga it is so important to look after yourself, to keep checking in, to keep listening to your own body and then to act accordingly. I believe it is important to try different styles, different approaches, different teachers, until you find what works for you – but then to keep checking in with this, because our needs inevitably change over time.

If you ignore your own feelings, bodily sensations and intuition, then you run the risk of engaging in mindless yoga, which is likely to result in some kind of injury. The important thing to focus on is what feels right for you.

MINDFUL YOGA EXERCISE

YOGA ASANA: STANDING FORWARD BEND (UTTANASANA)

This is a great posture for releasing tension in the hamstrings and lower back.

1. Start by standing in the middle of your mat with your feet hip-width apart, arms by your sides and shoulders relaxed.

2. Inhale as you lift your arms out to the sides and up above your head, with your thumbs gently touching.

3. As you exhale, start to slowly bend forwards from the pelvis. Keep your hips pushed back so that your buttocks stick out slightly.

4. Pause when you reach halfway, keeping a flat back. Inhale, then exhale and continue bending forwards as far as you are able.

5. If there is any pain in the lower back, or you have tight hamstrings, keep your knees bent slightly.

6. Take a few deep breaths and let everything hang. Your arms can dangle freely or you can hold onto your elbows. Slowly nod and shake the head a few times to release any tension.

7. You might want to bend one knee at a time to stretch the hamstrings. Or swing your torso from side to side. You can also slowly lift back up to the halfway position on an inhalation and release back down on an exhalation.

8. Breathe freely and move in a way that feels right for you, remembering to always do so with awareness.

9. When you are ready to come out, bend your knees, inhale and push through your feet, rolling up slowly with your chin tucked in and head coming up last. Roll your shoulders a few times when you reach the top.

Finding the Right Path for You

Working your way towards a more mindful yoga practice starts with finding your own path. It does not matter what others are doing, or what anyone else thinks you 'should' be doing; what matters is how you intuitively feel inside.

In my opinion, it is perfectly acceptable not to stick to one yoga style forever. Ashtanga was right for me then, but not now. It felt like it stopped working for me. It had become more of a pressure than a support in my life. Although I know it is possible to practise Ashtanga yoga mindfully, and I know many people who do, I found that I was unable to do this. I realized I was not practising mindfully and it felt like time to take a break. In the months that followed I found myself drawn to gentler, less rigid, styles of yoga, and I felt more in tune with what my body needed.

I will always be grateful for my Ashtanga practice. It helped me learn a lot about myself, it changed my lifestyle, and it made my body strong and flexible. But, as someone who has a tendency to be quite hard on myself, the strictness and discipline of the routine became quite a challenge for me. Finding a more gentle, mindful way to practise yoga has resulted in a much softer approach to the practice, and I find I can really appreciate the benefits of yoga now, without it feeling so rigid or pressured.

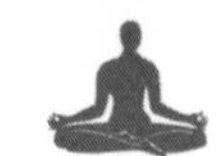

If you are a beginner, I would suggest your first step is to find the right teacher, even above finding the right yoga style. I have practised the same style of yoga with several different teachers and my experience has been vastly different. For me, the teacher has a huge impact on my overall experience of the practice, from the way they hold the space and give instructions, to the way they interact with me and talk about the practice. Every teacher is different and brings unique qualities to their teaching, but remember they should only act as a guide. Your yoga practice is yours alone, so you should feel in control of it.

It is important to follow your intuition, and you should always listen to your body rather than following a trend. By all means, try out the latest yoga style or go to the teacher that your friend recommends, but do not stick with it because of fashion or pressure – only because it feels right for you.

Your yoga practice is yours alone, so you should feel in control of it

Remember that what you need changes over time. Most of us are probably not into the same things we were into ten, or even five, years ago. Our interests change, our priorities change and our beliefs and value systems often change. It is the same with yoga. A style or teacher that really resonated with you two years ago might seem far less relevant now, and you might need something different. Perhaps you have more energy and want to try a more dynamic, flowing practice. Perhaps you feel the need for rest and relaxation and feel more attracted to restorative yoga styles. Or perhaps you merely feel curious and want to try something new.

In the final chapter we will bring together all the practices we have explored throughout this book into a seamless mindful yoga sequence. I would invite you to find your own path with this. By all means practise the sequence exactly as it is written, particularly if you are a beginner. For the more advanced yogi, you may wish to incorporate only certain elements of the mindful practices into your existing yoga practice. Above all, do what feels right for you and practise, practise, practise!

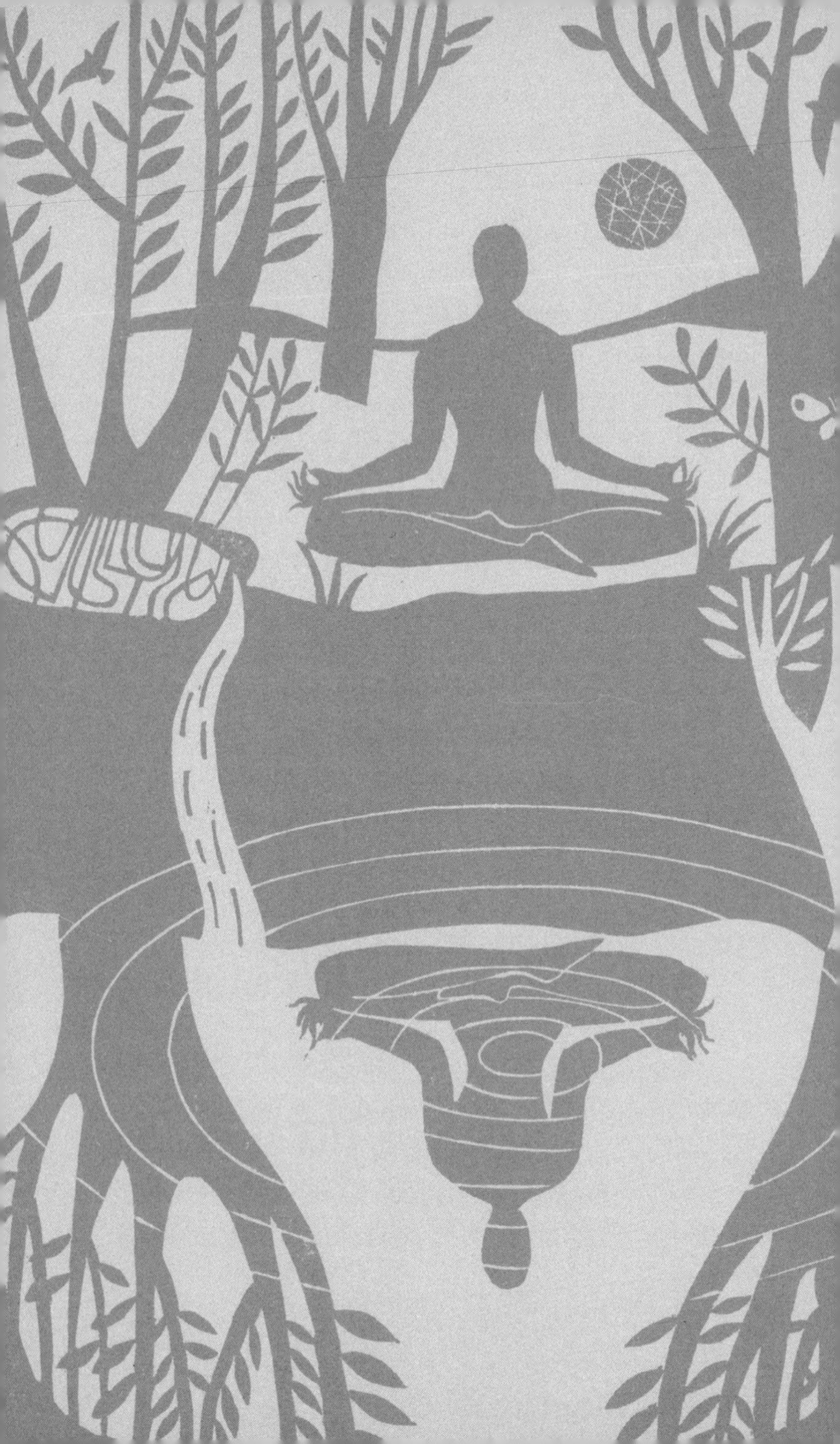

CHAPTER FIVE

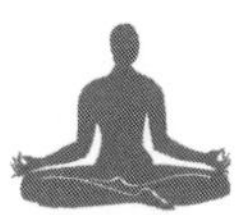

How to Practise Mindful Yoga

Practising mindful yoga is about listening to your body and trusting your intuition. Your body nearly always knows best; in fact, it usually knows a lot more than your mind does. You already have the answers; you simply need to tune in. Whether you are a beginner at yoga, or a more experienced practitioner, we will bring together everything we have learned so far into a connected practice of awareness – a sequence of mindful yoga.

Preparing for Practice

Before starting the mindful yoga sequence, I suggest reading the following guidelines for preparing your mind and body, so that you can stay completely present, with clarity, awareness and acceptance, throughout your entire practice.

Your body intuitively knows how it wants to move and what is best for it right now. You might want to follow a sequence you have followed before, drawing on experiences from different teachers and styles of yoga, or you might want to practise more spontaneously. Sometimes it can be helpful to start with a set sequence to get going (such as the one included in this chapter), and then move into a more spontaneous practice from there. The important thing is to listen to your body and move in a way that feels right for you in each moment. If you experience any sharp or shooting pain, you should stop immediately.

Listen to your body and move in a way that feels right for you in each moment

Remember: this is your practice. There are no prizes for achieving a 'perfect' posture; equally, there are no punishments for getting it 'wrong'. Asanas are not about making pretty shapes on the outside; it is how you feel on the inside that matters most. If you feel like holding a particular posture for a few minutes at a time, then do so. Or if you feel like being more fluid in a posture and bringing in gentle movements, then do this instead.

As long as your mind is calm and listening within, your breathing even, and all five senses alert, then you will be practising with full awareness – and when you are practising with full awareness, you will be completely grounded in the present moment. Out of this comes spontaneous, mindful movement. Once you are familiar with the routine and comfortable with incorporating the mindful practices, do feel free to explore and add in any other poses you like.

Above all, mindful yoga should be enjoyable. Sure, there might be times when it feels more challenging, or a certain ache or pain causes discomfort, but, generally speaking, I would encourage you to have fun with it. After all, if you are not enjoying yourself, then what is the point?

The three most important things to remember during any mindful yoga practice are:

- Focus on your breathing.
- Listen to your body.
- Trust your intuition.

Beginners

If you are a complete beginner, I would advise starting your asana practice with a good, experienced teacher, either at a class or online; there are plenty of online courses and tutorials available with reputable teachers. This will help you understand the fundamentals of yoga asana, how to safely move in and out of the postures, and about correct alignment in certain poses.

Once you have learned the basics, you can either start to practise mindful yoga at home or continue to attend classes, but bringing in mindful practices wherever you can.

When practising the sequence in this chapter, make sure you follow the instructions carefully, and listen to your body. If there is any 'bad' pain, stop immediately but carefully – do not suddenly wrench yourself out of the pose. Stay mindful. You will see the terms 'front' and 'back' in reference to your yoga mat. This simply refers to the short ends of the mat, dependent on your preference or position.

Mindful yoga is about how it feels, not how it looks

Remember, it is far more important to listen to yourself than to achieve the 'perfect' posture – mindful yoga is about how it feels, not how it looks.

Experienced Practitioners

If you are already an experienced yoga practitioner, learning to move in a more mindful way can have a hugely positive impact on your relationship with the practice. It can reveal all sorts of habits and behavioural patterns that you were not even aware of.

Try to move away from what you already know. Test out unfamiliar postures, or move into postures in a new way. If you always hold a static pose for a set amount of time, see what happens if you move slightly instead. If you always move to a certain depth in a posture because you know you can, what happens if you hold back? Or move more gradually towards that point? Sometimes we can feel muscles working or tension releasing that we would not otherwise have felt.

It can be so useful to recognize our habits and then purposefully change them. For example, I sometimes practise a posture the Ashtanga way because my body is so used to it. If I then bring more mindfulness to that posture, it often changes, and I find myself moving differently – usually more softly and with more awareness.

Mindful Movement

In mindful yoga, the postures are not there simply to be ticked off. Once you have moved into a posture, really embody it and be in it. How does it feel to be in this posture right now, to be making this shape with your body?

Moving mindfully in yoga is not just about how we get into the asanas; releasing out of them is just as important. You need to allow your body time to let go, to settle from the movements you just made. And this can be a slow process, particularly for more challenging postures, or if you have held a posture for a long time. We often practise a counter-pose after such postures to help rebalance and realign the body, and it can be important to let the body settle, even before moving into a counter-pose.

Trust the Niggles

Although I have said you should always listen to your body and do what feels right, sometimes there is a balance to be made. For example, it is not advisable to always avoid poses you do not like, as they are often the most useful. There is a fine line between an ache or pain that feels 'wrong' and one that just feels a bit 'niggly' or 'crunchy'. The niggles and crunch points are important, as they show us what needs working on. Learning to tell the difference is a crucial part of mindful yoga.

Follow your intuition, trust your instincts and embrace those niggly bits!

Your hips might feel a bit stiff or crunchy, because they need opening. You might experience burning thighs in certain postures, but this usually means they need strengthening. Your neck and shoulders might feel sore and stiff, simply because they are holding tension that needs releasing. Yoga can really help to ease, release, open and strengthen every part of our body – but only if we allow it to.

I believe each of us already knows which parts of ourselves need focusing on, so the crunch points serve as a reminder to draw our attention there more acutely. Follow your intuition, trust your instincts and embrace those niggly bits!

Mindful Yoga Sequence

The sequence outlined below is designed to guide you through a simple mindful yoga practice. Many of the poses include suggested mindful practices to be incorporated at the same time. As you become more familiar with the sequence, do feel free to add or remove postures and mix up the mindful practices as you prefer. Remember, this is ultimately a spontaneous practice, so listen to your body.

Some of the mindful practices introduced earlier can be used throughout your yoga practice whenever the need arises. These include:

- *Deep listening*. In this case to your body.
- *Labelling thoughts*. Whenever you notice your mind getting caught up in your thoughts, simply label what kind of thoughts they are and come back to your breath.
- *Using your breath to calm you down*. If you find yourself becoming anxious or agitated, or your breath quickens due to holding a challenging posture, simply take a few deeper breaths and focus on the air travelling in and out of your body.

Of course, it can be difficult to move mindfully while reading and following instructions at the same time. One way you could get around this is to practise with a friend or partner.

They can read the instructions to you as you practise and vice versa, until you become more familiar with the sequence. Alternatively, you could record yourself reading the instructions out loud, so you can then practise to the sound of your own voice.

Similar to preparing for a meditation, it is best to find a quiet place, free from distractions, where you will not be disturbed. Ensure there is enough space around your yoga mat to move without restriction. It does not matter whether you wear tight or loose-fitting clothes, as long as you can move easily and comfortably. To start with, you might want to wear a warmer layer, and perhaps keep your socks on if the room is cooler. You should remove the latter once you get moving, though, for a better grip and to avoid your feet slipping on the mat.

Find a quiet place, free from distractions, where you will not be disturbed

You can practise this sequence at any time of day. Personally, I prefer to do it first thing in the morning, before breakfast; however, many people feel too stiff at this time and prefer to stretch later in the day. Whatever time you practise, it is best to do so on an empty stomach, or at least an hour after a light meal or snack. If you are too full, you are likely to feel heavier on your mat, less comfortable in inverted postures, and more constricted in postures such as twists and forward bends.

You should allow thirty to forty-five minutes for the whole sequence, but this will vary depending on the amount of time you have available, the speed of your breath, and how long you choose to spend in each posture.

Warm-up

Easy Pose (Sukhasana)

Start by coming into Easy Pose, sitting cross-legged on your yoga mat. There should be a sufficient gap between your feet and pelvis so that a triangle shape is formed by your two thighs and crossed shins. You can use your hands to help arrange your buttocks, so that you can more easily feel your sitting bones on the mat. Your hands can rest in your lap or on your knees.

Despite its name, this asana can be challenging for many people, particularly if you are used to sitting in chairs or have knee problems. If your knees hurt, or do not comfortably release towards the floor, try putting a cushion or rolled-up blanket under them for support. If your spine is not upright, or you feel yourself slouching forwards, try sitting on a block or firm cushion to get more lift. Above all, make sure you are able to sit comfortably for a few minutes and that there is no pinching or sharp pain.

Take a few deep breaths to settle into the posture and fully arrive on your yoga mat. Check in with your body. How are you feeling? Are there any areas of tension? How is your mind? Is it calm or racing? And how is your breath? Take a few minutes to observe the breath, noticing how it feels as it travels in through your nose, all the way through your body and back out through your nose again. If you find your mind wandering, use an anchor for the breath (page 51). Pick the area where you feel it most – perhaps the edge of the nostrils, the back of the throat, the chest, ribs or stomach – and keep focusing on that area, bringing your attention back there each time it strays.

This is a wonderful opportunity to set your intention for your practice. Perhaps it is to let go of impatience or worries. Maybe it is to remain present and aware throughout. Or it could simply be to practise with complete acceptance, allowing for whatever needs to arise.

You might also choose to dedicate your practice to someone at this point. It could be a loved one, close friend, colleague, or even someone you do not know very well or are having difficulty with. You can simply bring them to mind and say silently to yourself that today you dedicate your practice to this person, and give a reason if it feels appropriate. This might be to send loving thoughts or healing prayers to them, or to help them with a challenge they are facing.

Cross-Legged Side Stretch

Once you are ready, take a breath in and stretch both arms straight up above your head. Then, as you exhale, take your right hand to the floor beside you, bending your right elbow slightly, and stretch your left arm up above over your head and over to the right as you stretch in that direction. Breathe. You should feel the stretch all the way up your left side. For a stronger stretch, bend the right elbow more deeply and stretch up further into the left fingertips.

On an exhalation, slowly return to a neutral position. Then inhale and repeat on the other side. Repeat once more on each side, stretching a little deeper each time, then slowly return to a neutral position.

Cross-Legged Twist

Take a breath in, stretching both arms straight up above your head again. As you exhale, take your right hand to the floor behind you, close to your buttocks. You can be up on your fingertips or with your palm flat to the floor, whichever is more comfortable. Place your left hand on your right knee and inhale as you lift your chest and straighten your spine. As you exhale, twist to the right, making sure you twist from your waist first – your head and neck should turn last. Breathe.

On each inhalation, see if you can lift up a little more, and on each exhalation, see if you can twist a little more. But do not force it; these should be subtle, mindful movements.

On an exhalation, return to the centre, then repeat on the other side. Repeat once more on each side, lifting and twisting a little deeper each time.

Cat-Cow Pose (Chakravakasana)

Now uncross your legs and gently move them round to one side so that you can come onto all fours on your hands and knees. Your shoulders should be aligned above your wrists and your hips should be aligned above your knees, so that you are making a square, box-like shape. Your gaze should be down towards the floor so that your neck is kept in a straight line with your spine.

As you inhale, start to lift your head and chest, dropping your belly button towards the floor and lifting your hips and buttocks up towards the ceiling, then gently tip your head back and look up (Cow Pose). As you exhale, start to lower your head and chest, rounding your back and sucking your belly button in towards your spine (Cat Pose). Only your spine should move during these poses; your arms and legs should remain stationary.

Keep repeating these two poses in a slow, flowing movement, inhaling as you lift your chest and exhaling as you round the back. See if you can feel your spine stretching and 'waking up' as you link the breath with the movement. After a few rounds, or when you are ready, slowly come back to a neutral, flat-back position and take a few breaths here.

Balancing Tabletop Pose (Dandayamana Bharmanasana)

From this position, inhale as you slowly lift your right arm and left leg off the ground. Extend your arm straight out in front of you and your leg straight behind you, and stretch through your fingers and toes. Your left toes should be pointed and your right thumb should be pointed upwards, with your palm facing to the left. Look down at your mat to keep your neck straight.

Take a few breaths here, then slowly release back to neutral and repeat on the other side. For a more intense stretch, you can also try bringing your extended arm and leg inwards, whilst rounding the back, so that the elbow and knee come towards each other; then extend out again. You will need to keep your gaze focused on a point on your mat in order to keep your balance.

Child's Pose (Balasana)

From a neutral all-fours position, inhale when you are ready. Then, as you exhale, start to move your hips backwards. You can either bring your knees and feet together so they are parallel, or you can bring your big toes towards each other and your knees out a little wider. Your buttocks should come to rest on top of your heels.

If your forehead reaches the floor, you can rest it there. If not, you can make two fists with your hands to rest your head on, or use a cushion or block. If you are not resting on your hands, your arms can either be stretched out on the mat in front of you, or you can bring them around behind you so that your hands rest near your feet, palms facing upwards.

Remember, it is more important that your buttocks are comfortably resting back on your heels than how far your head comes forward. Stay here for a few deep breaths.

You can introduce a simple breath counting exercise here. Inhale slowly through your nose whilst silently counting up to four; then gently hold your breath to the same count of four. Slowly exhale through your nose for a count of six, letting the air release steadily with control. Take a micro-pause at the end of the exhalation, then repeat for another four rounds. When you have finished, breathe normally for a few breaths to allow the body and mind to settle again.

Downward Dog (Adho Mukha Svanasana)
When you are ready, come out of Child's Pose by slowly lifting your head and chest until you are in a kneeling position. Take a breath here to allow your body to settle.

Now, move forwards onto all fours again, but with your hands further forward than your shoulders. Curl your toes under, take a breath in and, as you exhale, lift your knees off the ground, push back into your hips and straighten your legs as much as possible to come into Downward Dog. Your hands should be shoulder-width apart and your feet hip-width apart. Breathe.

You can either remain in stillness here, or move in any way your body feels like moving. You might want to 'walk your dog' by bending one knee at a time to stretch the hamstrings, or come right up onto your toes, then push back down again through your heels. You could also lift one leg off the ground and stretch it up and behind you, or you might want to experiment by turning the elbows in and out and stretching through the shoulders.

This is a great asana for cultivating awareness, listening to your body and moving into those niggles (page 112). If the posture feels very strong on your hamstrings, or any other part of your body, you can always come back down into Child's Pose for a few breaths, then push back up into Downward Dog. You can do this as many times as you need to.

Remember not to worry about your heels reaching the ground in this posture, especially if you are a beginner. It can take years of daily practice for your heels to touch the ground – if at all – and it is more important to focus on getting a good stretch through your shoulders, hamstrings and calves.

Standing Forward Bend (Uttanasana)

Once you have had a good stretch in Downward Dog, walk your feet in towards your hands so that you come into a forward bend. Keep your feet hip-distance apart and your knees slightly bent. If there is any pain in your lower back, bend your knees more.

You can either let your arms and hands hang – whether they reach the floor or not – or you might want to hold opposite elbows and let your arms hang that way. Make sure you are not holding tension in your head and neck: let them hang freely. You can gently shake your head up and down and side to side to encourage this.

This posture should feel quite releasing. Keep your knees bent if you feel pain or stiffness in the lower back. You can try gently straightening one knee at a time to stretch the hamstrings. You can also try swinging from one side to the other so that you feel a bit like a rag doll, which can be a wonderful tension reliever.

To come out of the pose, start inhaling as you bend your knees deeply, push up through your feet and thighs, and slowly straighten your body. While coming up, keep a slight bend in your knees and your chin tucked into your chest; your head should come up last. Once fully upright, exhale and then roll your shoulders a couple of times to release them – first in one direction, then in the other. Take a few breaths here to allow your body to settle.

Mountain Pose (Tadasana)

Step to the front of your mat with your feet together. If your feet do not meet, they can stay a few inches apart, or hip-width apart if you prefer. Your legs should be straight, but with soft knees, not locked. Try to spread your toes apart as much as you can. Tuck your tailbone in slightly, so there is a natural curve in your lower back but your buttocks are not sticking out. Take your shoulders down and back, away from your ears. Your arms should rest a small distance away from your body with your palms facing slightly forwards. Your neck should sit straight on your spine, so you may need to tuck in your chin slightly.

Now, close your eyes and imagine there is a cord running all the way from the ground, up through your body and out through the top of your head. An invisible force is pulling the cord from the top, which subtly lifts your whole body upwards in a straight line.

Focus on your breathing and check in with your body. How are you feeling now you have completed this warm-up sequence? Do you feel more energized? Has some of the tension released? Stay here for a few breaths, or longer if you prefer, then slowly open your eyes again.

Standing Sequence

Triangle (Trikonasana)

From Mountain Pose, step back with your right foot and swivel your hips to the right to come into a medium wide-legged stance along your mat. Start with your feet parallel, roughly three to four foot lengths apart, so they are in line with the short edges of your mat. Raise your arms so they are also out to the sides.

Then, turn your left foot in slightly and turn your right foot out ninety degrees so that it is now parallel with the long edge of your mat. Make sure the heel of your right foot is in line with the arch of your left foot. Your hips should be squared forwards, pointing towards the long edge of your mat, with your eyes looking the same way.

Now turn your head to look along your right arm and inhale. As you exhale, reach into your right arm and shoulder and keep extending through the arm until you cannot reach any further. Then simply 'windmill' your arms so that your right hand drops to your right leg and your left arm lifts up in the air. It does not matter where your right hand lands – shin, ankle, foot or toe – as long as you are not putting pressure directly on your knee. Your arms should create a straight line.

Think about a person in your life for whom you are truly grateful

If it is comfortable for your neck, you can now turn your head to look up at your left hand. Breathe. And here you can practise some gratitude. Think about a person in your life for whom you are truly grateful, and see how it feels in your body. As you focus on this person, and embody this posture whilst breathing deeply, you might find yourself breaking into a gentle smile.

When you are ready, turn your head to look down at the floor, then inhale, push through your thighs and slowly lift out of the posture. Turn your feet back to the front and take a breath or two here. You can lower your arms if you need to. Then repeat on the other side.

This time, bring to mind something in your life for which you are grateful. It could be significant, such as having a roof over your head or the skills to do your job, or it could be simpler, such as the view from your window or a type of food that you love. Again, focus on this while you breathe and relax into the posture. Come out slowly when you are ready and return to the front of your mat.

Warrior One (Virabhadrasana I)

Step out to the side again with your right foot, but this time take your feet slightly wider apart. Start with your feet parallel and your hands on your hips. Now turn your left foot in slightly and your right foot out ninety degrees, as you did for Triangle, but this time turn your hips so they are facing towards your right foot. You should now be facing the short edge of your mat. Try to get your hips square, so focus on encouraging your right hip to move backwards and your left hip forwards. You might need to turn the left foot in a little more. Check that your right heel is still in line with the arch of your left foot.

Now slowly bend your right knee so that your right thigh sinks towards the floor. Make sure your right knee does not extend over your right ankle. If it does, adjust your feet so they are slightly wider apart. Sink down through the hips as much as possible. Then, inhale, take your arms up above your head with your palms facing each other and look up towards

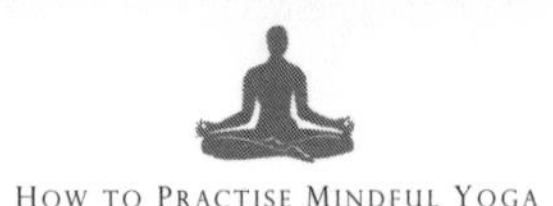

your hands. Sink your hips down, stretch your arms up and breathe. You are now in Warrior One.

It is great to practise some positive affirmations while you are in such a strong, powerful posture. These are short phrases in the present tense encompassing beliefs, behaviours and personality traits that you have or would like to have, for example: 'I am a beautiful, creative being', 'I am truly loved', or 'I am enough and I have all that I need.'

On your next inhalation, push through your thighs to straighten your right leg and swivel around to the other side, keeping your arms stretched up above your head. Check the alignment of your feet, then exhale and bend the left leg to repeat the pose on this side. This time choose another affirmation to say silently to yourself whilst you sink into the posture and breathe. Rather than coming back to centre, go straight into the next posture from here.

Warrior Two (Virabhadrasana II)

From Warrior One, you can open straight out into Warrior Two. Inhale as you take your arms down and out to the sides, square your hips in line with the long edge of your mat and look along your left arm. Remember to keep your arms straight, your thighs strong and your hips sinking down. Do not let your left knee extend over your left ankle.

Here, you can practise the first stage of the Loving Kindness meditation, repeating this simple mantra silently to yourself:

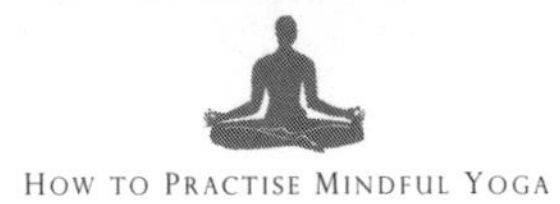

May I be happy.

May I be healthy.

May I be free from all suffering.

May I be peaceful and at ease.

Really focus on each phrase of the mantra, sending these loving intentions to yourself. Feel the power of the posture as you do so.

On your next inhalation, straighten your left leg and swivel yourself around to the other side. Then, as you exhale, bend your right knee and look along your right arm. Breathe deeply and repeat your Loving Kindness mantra again.

When you are ready, inhale to come back to centre with your hands on your hips, exhale here, then step to the front of your mat.

Side Angle Pose (Utthita Parsvakonasana)

From here, step out to the side again with your right foot so that your feet are about the same distance apart as they were for Warrior One and Two. Again, turn your left foot in slightly and your right foot out ninety degrees. Make sure the heel of your right foot is in line with the arch of your left. Your hips should be squared to the long edge of your mat, with your hands on your hips.

Inhale and, as you exhale, bend your right knee and sink your hips towards the floor. Make sure your knee does not extend further than your ankle; adjust your feet wider if it does.

Then take your right elbow and rest it on your right knee. Try not to put all your weight into this elbow, but keep both thighs strong. Inhale, stretching your left arm up and over your head, so that it forms a straight line all the way up the left side of your body. Look up to your left hand if it is comfortable to do so in the neck. Exhale and relax into the posture. Keep breathing.

While in this posture, you can come back to your gratitude practice again. This time, think of something that happened this week for which you are thankful. Perhaps you received a nice compliment or someone cooked you a tasty meal.

On an inhalation, take your left arm back down and push up through the thighs to lift yourself back up, turning your feet back to the front. Exhale here, then repeat on the other side. This time, bring to mind something that happened today for which you are thankful. Even if you have not been up long, you might be grateful for the dreams you had in the night, the daylight filling the room or the hot drink you just enjoyed. Pleasure can be found even in the simplest moments of life.

When you are ready, inhale, come back to centre, then exhale and return to the front of your mat.

Wide-Legged Forward Bend (Prasarita Padottanasana)
Step out again with your right foot into a wide-legged stance. Keep your feet parallel, pointing towards the long edge of your mat, then turn the toes of both feet in a little. Put your

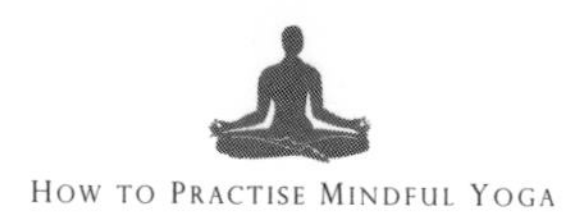

hands on your hips and tuck your tailbone in slightly. Inhale and lift your chest, then, as you exhale, start to hinge forwards from the hips. Move slowly and stop when you get halfway, where your back comes into parallel with the floor. Look towards the floor, so your neck is straight, then bring your hands down. You might come to your fingertips, or with your palms on the floor, depending on the length of your arms.

Feel the strength of your body as you embody your affirmations

Take a breath here. Then, on your next exhalation, hinge forwards a little more if you can, while bending in the elbows. Try to keep your hips and thighs pushing back, so that you are not tipping forwards. Your hands should be touching the floor now, with your elbows bent as much as they need to. If you cannot reach the floor with your hands, you can rest them on your legs, or use a yoga block or even a stack of books to lean on, but make sure your legs are bearing most of your weight. Your head and neck should hang freely. Keep breathing.

Here you can practise another positive affirmation. Bring to mind a positive statement, such as 'I have the energy and motivation to achieve whatever I desire', or 'I am a free-thinking individual with unique qualities', or 'I meet each new day with positivity and confidence'. Feel the strength of your body in this posture – especially in your thighs – as you embody your affirmations.

If you want to move in this pose, you can try gently swinging your torso and arms across towards one foot, then the other. You can try moving your hands further forward or back on the floor to see how this affects the stretch. Or you can gently lift up to the flat-back position, then release down again a few times.

When you are ready to come out, inhale as you come half-way up to the flat-back position with your fingertips on the floor, then exhale here as you place your hands on your hips. Inhale again to come all the way up, pushing through your feet and thighs. Then walk your feet in together and step to the front of your mat.

Tree Pose (Vriksasana)

Balancing postures are very good for cultivating mindfulness, as you cannot do anything but remain present in order to keep your balance.

Start by standing with your feet together at the front of your mat. Then shift your weight onto your left foot and turn your right hip out slightly, with your toes still on the floor and your right heel resting gently against your left ankle. If this feels enough, you can stay here. Focus your gaze on a point just in front of you to help keep your balance.

If you feel well balanced here, try taking your right foot higher, so that it rests against your left shin. Or, you can try taking it up to the thigh, but avoid resting it against the knee.

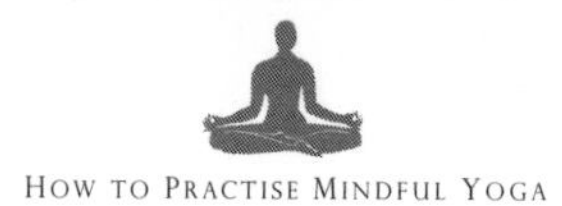

You can also use your hand to help move your right foot to the very top of your left inner thigh, so your heel almost meets your groin. Press your right foot and left thigh firmly against each other for more stability.

Wherever your foot is rested, once you have your balance here, you can bring your hands into prayer position in front of your sternum, or lift them up above your head with the palms pressed together. Keep your attention focused on a single point in front of you, and remember to breathe slowly and deeply. And smile!

For the ultimate test, you can try closing your eyes, even for a few seconds, and see if you can still keep your balance. This takes focus, concentration and complete presence.

When you are ready, gently release your arms, release your right foot and come back to standing. Then, repeat on the other side.

Chair Pose (Utkatasana)

Again, start by standing with your feet together at the front of your mat. Then inhale and lift your arms straight up above your head, with the palms facing each other, shoulder-width apart. As you exhale, slowly bend your knees, keeping the buttocks sticking out, as if you are about to sit down in a chair. Bend as low as you can and hover here, keeping the thighs strong to protect the knees, and looking straight ahead or slightly upwards towards your hands. Breathe.

You can now practise the second stage of the Loving Kindness meditation. So, bring to mind a loved one – it could be the person you dedicated your practice to, or someone else – and repeat this mantra to them:

May you be happy.

May you be healthy.

May you be free from all suffering.

May you be peaceful and at ease.

Focus all your attention on this person, strongly sending these loving intentions to them. Feel the power of the posture as you do so. Your thighs might be burning a little at this point!

To come out, inhale as you straighten up with your arms still raised, then exhale as you release your arms out wide and down to your sides. Take a few breaths here and allow your body to settle again.

Floor Sequence

Seated Forward Bend (Paschimottanasana)

Come down to a seated position in the middle of your mat with your legs straight out in front of you. You might want to shake, roll or pat down your legs to help them release from the strong standing postures. Lift each buttock with your hands, so that you can more easily feel your sitting bones on the floor, and keep your spine as upright as possible.

Inhale and lift your arms straight up above your head with your palms facing forwards. Keep your shoulders moving down away from your ears and lift your chest. As you exhale, start hinging forwards from the hips. It is a good idea to move very slowly and take as many breaths as you need. Remember, the point here is not to collapse, so focus on moving forwards rather than downwards. Keep your chest lifted and let gravity do most of the work. On each inhalation, lift your chest a little more; on each exhalation, see if you can move forwards a little further.

Bring to mind a person and repeat the mantra, sending them your well wishes

Wherever you get to, you can rest your hands on or beside your legs and let your head hang forwards. You might have only bent forwards a little way, or your head might be resting on your shins. What matters is that you are comfortable. If there is any pain in the lower back, you can bend your knees a little to relieve this.

Once you are comfortable, you can practise the third stage of Loving Kindness. Bring to mind a neutral person and repeat the mantra, sending them your well wishes:

May you be happy.

May you be healthy.

May you be free from all suffering.

May you be peaceful and at ease.

To come out of the posture, inhale as you slowly push yourself up, bringing your head up last.

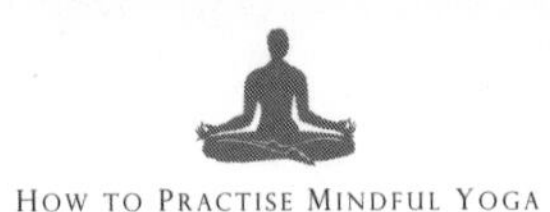

Seated Spinal Twist (Ardha Matsyendrasana)
From this seated position, bend your right knee and bring your foot flat to the floor so it is close to the groin. Now lift your right foot off the floor, cross it over your left knee and place it on the floor beside that knee. Wrap your left arm around the bent leg and hold the outside of your knee or thigh with your left hand. Inhale, place your right hand on the mat behind you, close to your buttocks, and lift your chest.

As you exhale, slowly twist to the right, starting from the waist and bringing your head around last. On each inhalation, lift your chest and straighten your spine a little more; on each exhalation, twist to the right a little more.

On your last exhalation, slowly twist back to the front, straighten out your legs and take a few breaths to allow your body to settle. Then repeat on the other side.

Cobra Pose (Bhujangasana)
From here, shift your weight to one side, bend your knees and bring your legs around and behind you, then come to lie down on your front. Your arms should be down by your sides, with your forehead to the floor or your head to the side resting on one cheek. Your toes should be pointed, not curled under. Take a few breaths here.

With your forehead to the floor, bring your hands up to shoulder level with your palms face down on the mat. Inhale and gently push through your hands to lift your head and chest off the floor with your chin tucked in, keeping your elbows bent and tucked in. Your thighs should be together, with your toes pressing down and back. Keep your chest lifted and look up, but do not tip your head right back. Try not to clench your buttocks.

If this feels like enough, stay here. If you can go further, you can try slowly straightening your arms for a deeper backbend. Only go as far as you are able and move mindfully. If there is any pain in your lower back, come down again.

Whichever level you lift up to, keep breathing deeply and evenly. When you are ready, gently release out of the posture on an exhalation.

Knee to Chest Pose (Apanasana)

Roll over onto your back with your legs outstretched. Keeping your left leg straight, bend your right knee off the floor, clasp both hands around it and 'hug' it into your chest. Take a few breaths here, then straighten it out again and repeat with the left leg.

You might want to take some time here for additional spine releasing movements. Try hugging both knees into your chest and gently rocking from side to side, or in little circles, to massage the spine. You can also make big circles with the knees, moving them away from each other, then back together, to release the hips. Remember to circle them in the opposite direction too. And keep breathing.

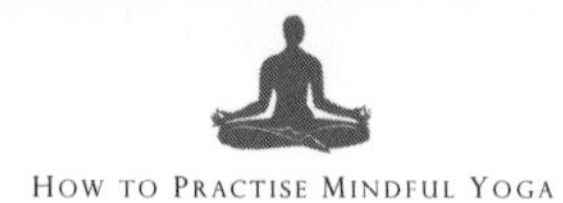

Gluteal Stretch

Stay lying on your back, bend both knees and bring your feet flat to the floor, close to your buttocks. Then lift your right foot off the ground and rest your right ankle on your left knee, so that your right hip is turned outwards slightly. Lift your left foot off the floor and clasp both hands around your left thigh. You should feel a stretch in your right glutes, i.e. in the buttocks and down the back of the thigh. If not, gently pull the thigh in closer towards your chest for a stronger stretch. After a few breaths, return both feet to the floor and repeat on the other side.

Supine Spinal Twist (Supta Jathara Parivartanasana)

Whilst still lying on your back, start with both knees bent, feet flat on the floor, and arms out to the sides at shoulder height. Inhale and lift both feet off the floor, bring your knees towards your chest slightly, then exhale as you slowly move them over to the right side and towards the floor. They may not reach the floor, and you can use your right hand to gently encourage them down if that feels comfortable. Turn your head to the left.

You might find that you cannot get both your knees and your left shoulder fully to the floor at the same time. You can play with this by gently rocking between your knees and shoulder; you should feel a nice releasing sensation in your back as you do so.

Whilst in this posture, you can practise the final stage of Loving Kindness, directing your mantra towards someone you have difficulty with:

May you be happy.

May you be healthy.

May you be free from all suffering.

May you be peaceful and at ease.

If it is too difficult to imagine saying your mantra directly to them, you can recite your mantra in the third person: 'May [name] be happy', 'May [name] be healthy', and so on.

When you are ready, inhale to come back to centre, then repeat on the other side. You can repeat any of the Loving Kindness stages here, or simply focus on your breath.

Finishing Sequence

Corpse Pose (Shavasana)

For the final relaxation pose, remain lying on your back with your eyes closed and arms by your sides, palms facing upwards, a little way out from your body. You can roll your shoulder blades back and slightly underneath you to bring the shoulders away from the ears. If there is tension in your lower back, you might prefer to keep your knees bent with your feet flat on the floor. Otherwise, extend your legs out straight, a little way apart, and let your feet flop out to the sides.

Your chin should be slightly tucked in; you might want a folded blanket or thin cushion under your head for support.

You can also place a bolster, cushion or rolled up blanket under your knees, if your legs are extended.

You can stay in Shavasana for anything from five to twenty minutes, depending on the time you have available, so make sure you are warm and comfortable. You might want to put on socks and another layer, or cover yourself in a blanket. You could also use an eye pillow to block out any harsh light.

Let any controlled breathing go and remain still

Take a few deep breaths to help settle your body, and try to relax fully into the mat. Then let any controlled breathing go and remain still and quiet.

If you find yourself getting easily distracted, try one of the mindfulness practices, such as focusing on sounds (page 82) or finding an anchor for the breath (page 51), or repeat any of the affirmations, gratitude or Loving Kindness practices you followed during your mindful yoga sequence. Another good practice to do whilst lying down is the body scan (page 80). Take some time to scan through your whole body, from the head to the toes, bringing your awareness to each part in turn and seeing if you can relax that part just a little bit more.

When you are ready to come out, it is important to do so slowly and gently. Start to wriggle the fingers and toes first, then stretch out in any way that feels right for you. Then, with your eyes still closed, slowly roll over onto one side and take

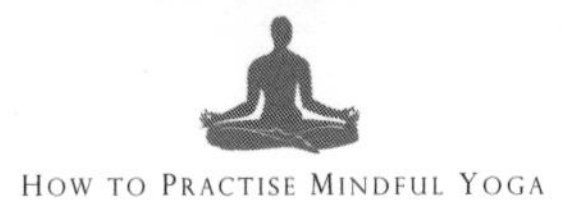

a few breaths here. On an inhalation, push yourself up using your hands and come to a cross-legged or other comfortable seated position on your mat.

Closing the Practice

If you have time, I would recommend practising a short meditation here, perhaps ten to fifteen minutes, as it is a wonderful way to round off your mindful yoga sequence. It is usually best to practise meditation after yoga, because it is easier to sit for a prolonged period once you have moved and stretched your body first. You can listen to a guided meditation, or follow a meditation practice, for example, counting the breath (page 50) or the mindfulness of breathing (page 53). Or simply sit and just be.

You can close your practice any way you choose. Many group classes end by chanting three long Oms together. As we saw in chapter one, Om is a way of saying yes to everything, so it is a very positive way to end your mindful yoga practice. You can chant your Oms out loud or in your head, whichever feels more appropriate.

At the end of my own practice, I like to bring my hands into the prayer position and silently recite my own prayer. This gives thanks to my Angels, the Universe, the Sun and the Moon, and invokes positivity and confidence into my day. I then say *Namaste* (a respectful Hindi greeting), bow down and touch the earth to give thanks.

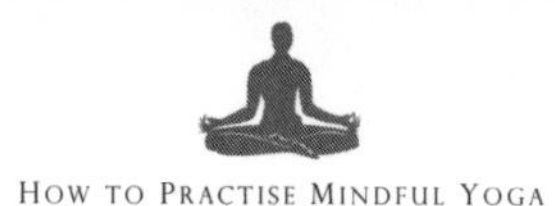

How Do You Feel?

Now that you have practised a mindful yoga sequence, how are you feeling? Did you enjoy bringing more awareness to your practice? How did you find the integration of mindful practices with yoga asanas? Were you able to listen to your body more? Did you allow your body to lead your mind, rather than the other way around?

I hope that the ideas and suggestions presented in this book inspire you to practise yoga in a more mindful way, thereby encouraging more acceptance and compassion into other areas of your life. In my experience, a mindful life is a happy one and I am sure you would agree that we could all do with a little more happiness in our lives.

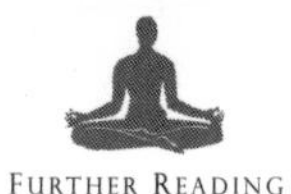

FURTHER READING

Bryant, Edwin F., *The Yoga Sutras of Patañjali*, New York, North Point Press, 2009

Kabat-Zinn, Jon, *Full Catastrophe Living: How to Cope with Stress, Pain and Illness Using Mindfulness Meditation*, London, Little, Brown Book Group, revised edition 2013

Rosenberg, Marshall B., *Nonviolent Communication: A Language of Life*, California, PuddleDancer Press, 2003

Sweet, Corinne, *The Mindfulness Journal: Exercises to Help You Find Peace and Calm Wherever You Are*, London, Boxtree, 2014

Yoga Journal and Yoga Alliance in partnership with Ipsos Public Affairs, *2016 Yoga in America Study*, January 2016 <http://media.yogajournal.com/wp-content/uploads/2016-Yoga-in-America-Study-Topline-RESULTS.pdf>

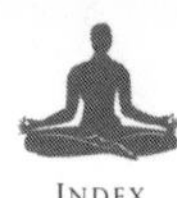

INDEX

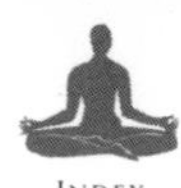

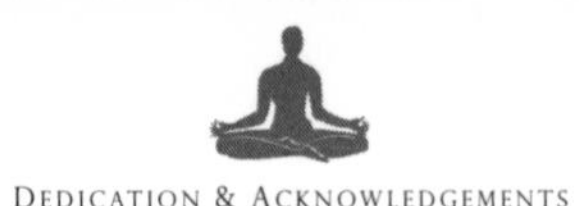

Dedication

This book is dedicated to my mother, Mumukshu, without whom I might never have taken my first step into a yoga class. She continues to be the strongest source of love and inspiration in my life.

Acknowledgements

I would like to thank all of my yoga, meditation and mindfulness teachers, both past and present, for their wisdom, their unending encouragement and support, and their unwavering faith in the process.

I would also like to thank everyone at Leaping Hare Press for allowing me the opportunity to write my first book. A special thank you goes to Monica Perdoni for her support and to Tom Kitch and Elizabeth Clinton for putting up with my endless barrage of questions.

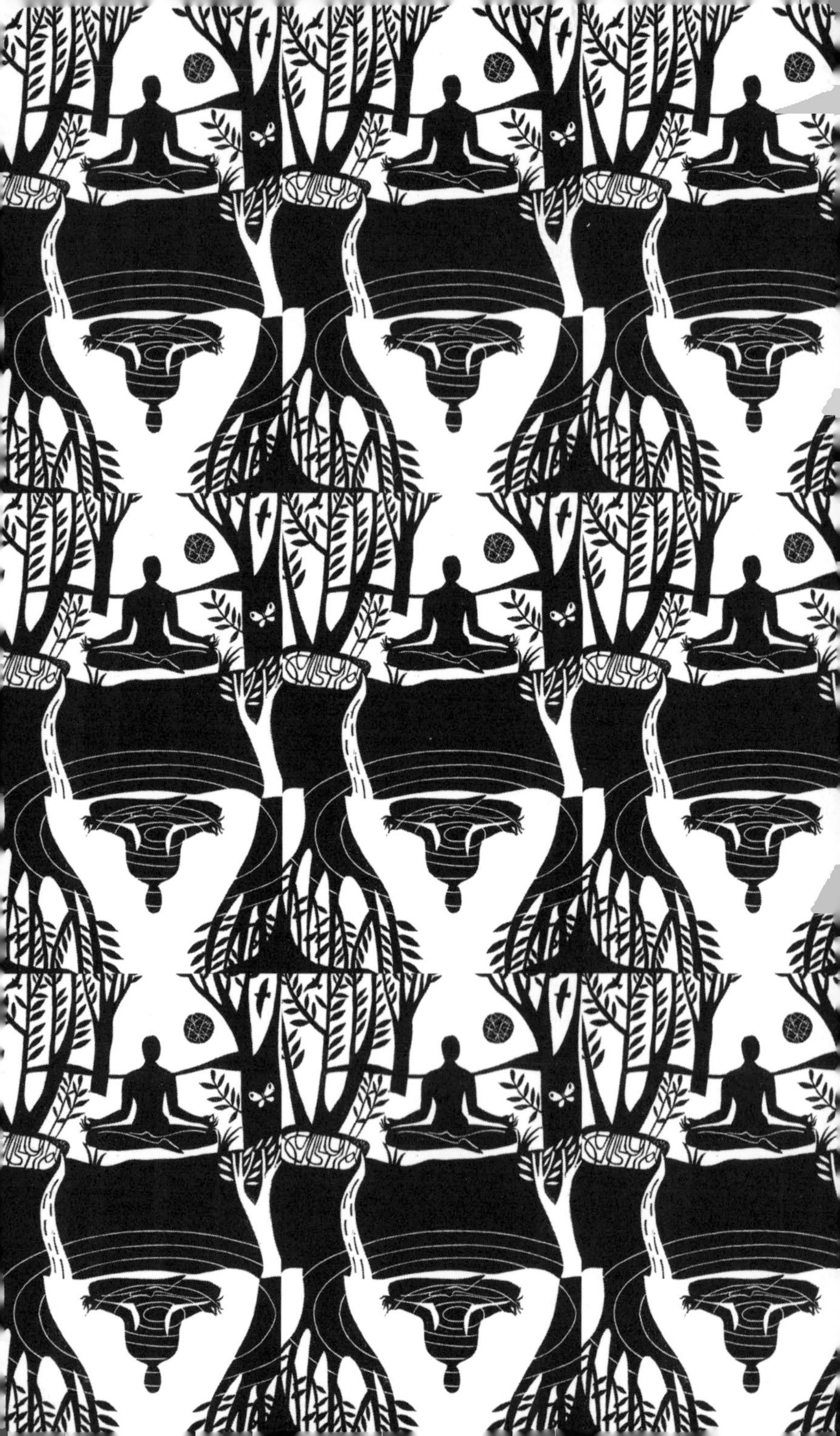